THE POWER

OF RARE

———

PRAISE FOR *THE POWER OF RARE*

"I don't read books, I'm way too busy for that, but if I did I'd read this one. Victoria Jackson is one of my closest friends and one smart strong woman. Even when she texts me I read it over and over again because it's so well written. So I feel I can say with 100% confidence if you read this book you will learn something and see why I love and admire her so much."
—Ellen DeGeneres

"I have watched for a decade as Victoria Jackson has been funding and creating circles instead of hierarchies and has brought a new and unprecedented collaboration between NMO researchers, drug companies not prone to collaboration, and otherwise isolated patients."
—Gloria Steinem

"This is an important story about a mother's push to transform the world of biomedical research. Victoria Jackson's book is a reminder that power lives all around us, often in the most unlikely places."
—Maria Shriver

"I once said that it takes either desperation or inspiration to transform vision into reality. *The Power of Rare* is the gripping story of how Victoria Jackson drew from the desperation to save her daughter from a life-threatening illness and used inspiration to create a revolutionary blueprint for curing rare and common diseases alike."
—Tony Robbins

"Victoria Jackson has been an endless source of inspiration to me. Through the power of a mother's love she has transformed the competitive world of medical research. I'm so glad she has shared her blueprint in *The Power of Rare* so more people can benefit from her tireless efforts."
—Reese Witherspoon

"*The Power of Rare* is as much a book about rare leadership as it is a true story of how one mother, with no background in health or medicine, has built a global movement to cure a life-threatening rare disease that impacts every nation of this earth. Her blueprint should be studied by all leaders as we come together to solve all diseases—rare and common alike."
—Ibrahim Boubacar Keïta,
President of the Republic of Mali

"*The Power of Rare* is an important story of how dedication and passion for the love of a child coupled with the drive, ingenuity and generosity of a rare individual, namely Victoria Jackson, can change the medical paradigm to break down silos and enhance collaboration in a race toward a cure. It's a great read and a story that needs to be told to inspire others."
—Robin L. Smith, MD, MBA,
Chairman and President of
The Stem for Life Foundation

"Victoria Jackson is an innovative entrepreneur, and an iconoclast. *The Power of Rare* tells the against-all-odds story of how this remarkable leader used her passion and raw determination to revolutionize medical research. The profound effects of her accomplishments will inspire all who strive to make a difference in the world."
—Greg Renker,
Founding Principal and Co-Chairman,
Guthy|Renker

"As you read *The Power of Rare*, you'll be moved to the depths of gratitude by how Victoria Jackson has demonstrated for all of us the incredible resourcefulness for doing whatever life calls you to do. She has given us all a profound gift of knowing that the impossible is absolutely possible."
—Agapi Stassinopoulos,
Author of *Wake Up To The Joy of You*

"Nine years ago, almost nothing was known about NMO, a rare disease we now understand afflicts tens of thousands across the African continent. Thanks to the life-saving work led by Victoria Jackson to cure NMO, there is great hope for improving and saving lives—and for solving other diseases that are not so rare."
—Professor Samba Sow,
Minister of Health and Public Hygiene, Mali

"*The Power of Rare* is a gift for patients, caregivers, clinicians, and scientists alike who seek answers and solutions to the growing epidemic of rare, autoimmune, and other diseases that impact the entire world. Ms. Jackson's call to action for a revolution in caring about rare and each other is a message whose time has come."
—Professor Mansour Ndiaye,
Président African Academy of Neurology: AFAN

THE POWER OF RARE

A BLUEPRINT FOR
A MEDICAL REVOLUTION

VICTORIA JACKSON

WITH

DR. MICHAEL YEAMAN

To my beautiful daughter Ali

In the midst of winter,

I found there was within me

an invincible summer.
—*Albert Camus*

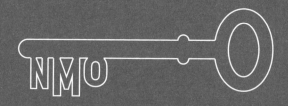

CONTENTS

REDEFINING RARE

The value of rare is something I appreciate, something I know intuitively in my life. And the recognition that each of us is infinitely unique—truly rare—is one of those simple, enduring truths that has long spoken to me.

Growing up, I remember secretly thinking of myself as someone who was too different, who didn't quite fit in. An outsider. But over the years I've come to embrace and feel empowered by my rare identity. I've also always been most attracted to those who dare to be rare—who think differently, who don't follow form or fashion but who celebrate the very qualities that set them apart.

The more I've studied rare, the more I've chosen to honor how unique every single human being is—each life is. Not just our faces and fingerprints but our stories and our struggles and our dreams. Yet what I've learned in recent years is that even though most everyone can agree about this universal aspect of rare, it raises one of the greatest challenges in modern medicine: if each of us is fundamentally unique, then why are so many treated with the exact same medicine?

Less than a decade ago, such a thought probably would not have been a concern. Much less something I'd be able to articulate.

Fast-forward. This very provocative question had somehow delivered me to a James Bond, 007–themed conference room at Google headquarters in Silicon Valley, California. I was there to make a presentation to some of the most tech-savvy executives around—and to ask them to turn their supercomputer powers from digital codes to disease cures. Sitting there waiting for them to arrive, I couldn't help but imagine these techies walking in the room as thirty-something hyper-achievers ironically wearing hoodies and lugging backpack laptops.

And so they did—as if in uniform.

I jokingly said, "You know I really feel like I'm in the middle of an episode of *Silicon Valley*," referring to the image of the characters on the TV show and their laid-back lifestyle as "disrupters"—to use their lingo—who are creating the future.

One of the more serious young execs said, "We don't consider that show a sitcom. It's a documentary."

Silence. Then everyone turned to me and waited to hear what I was there to say.

Deep breath.

There have been so many surreal moments on my current journey when I've had to ask myself, *How did I get here, and why did the universe choose me for this path?* This was definitely one of those moments. Not so many years earlier, talking to such brainiacs about Big Data and its use in medical research would have been as likely as me being invited to speak at the Vatican about new cures for an autoimmune disease. And as the universe would have it, both of these impossible moments—and many others—have come true in the course of a lifeline that has taken me from mascara to medicine.

True. The fact is that until February 2008, my professional expertise and success came from making and marketing cosmetics. From lip gloss to moisturizer—these were my tools of the trade for a larger vision. One, in retrospect, that has many parallels to curing a rare disease. I could see the unique beauty in each woman and knew a way to reveal it from the inside out. I was passionate about helping women feel better about themselves and their lives—and wanted to share what I knew.

Going against the old rules of the cosmetics business, I followed the guidance of my own intuition to create change. That intuitive capacity is sometimes hard to explain; somehow, I understood how to bring the innate beauty in others to the surface. Even so, before I became a makeup artist–turned–cosmetics entrepreneur who challenged the status quo of the beauty world, I was a high school dropout who never dreamed of being able to attend a college class.

Since those early days, I've been amazingly fortunate that my life experiences and challenges have helped make up for my lack of formal education. Besides earning what has amounted to a doctorate in "street smarts," I long ago learned the value of self-education—at every stage of life. Still, I'm the first to admit that my choice to give up mascara for medicine was not made because I was by any means the best candidate for doing so. No, this choice to take a real-life crash course in everything one needs to know to solve a rare autoimmune disease was made out of desperation, anguish, and absolute necessity. My self-taught medical school began the day my beautiful fourteen-year-old daughter, Ali, was diagnosed with a rare, life-threatening, and terrifying "orphan" condition called neuromyelitis optica, or NMO. And when I realized how poorly understood this disease was—and that there were few treatments and no cures—every day became devoted to changing that reality.

The same capacity for harnessing intuition that I used as an entrepreneur has served me well on the journey to curing NMO.

We hear the term "rare" so often that it's almost a cliché—until you look at it in a different light. The chance of being struck by lightning in a given year is about 1 in a million. Rare. However, the chance of being struck by lightning in any one lifetime is about 1 in 10,000. Not so rare after all. And even more relatable, everyone understands what lightning is, can read the signs to predict it, and knows to respect it. If only the same were true for rare diseases like NMO.

Then how rare—really—is this rare disease with its misleading, simple three-letter name? Today, based on our work that has taken on this would-be killer, researchers have refined their estimates to suggest that it may impact as many as 500,000 people worldwide. Not so different from the prevalence of lightning strikes; such numbers nearly equal 1 in 10,000. But back in 2008—in those dark and frightening early hours of this journey—I remember hearing that only 2,000 patients in the world had NMO.

Such extreme odds fit into a recurring theme in my life—what I call the Rule of 2%. As far back as I can remember, when faced with the most unlikely of odds for something happening, that is exactly what would happen to me. The awareness crystallized for me several years ago when I was at the dentist and asked what to expect about a procedure and how long it would take to recuperate.

"Most people do fine," he said. "But there's always that 2%." Turns out, he said, a tiny percentage of patients have had unique challenges that could make the process more difficult.

I knew then and there that's where I'd be—in the 2%. Yep, and I told the dentist so.

He laughed.

During the procedure, there were a few surprises, and he had to agree: "You know, you're right. You are one of the 2%."

This may seem like a mundane example, but after that experience and countless like it in my life, I started referring to these rare events as my personal Rule of 2%.

Sometimes the 2% can be bad. But sometimes it can be good—like amazingly good. It's the Rule that wins the lottery . . . that helps you turn crazy pipedream ideas into ways to revolutionize the marketplace . . . and, yes, it was the very Rule that once empowered a scared, insecure but determined teenager (me) to eventually build a cosmetics empire. Somehow my Rule turned a struggling young, then-single mom into a global Good Will Ambassador for Mascara. The Rule of 2% can turn the impossible into the possible, and brings with it the capability of empowering and transforming other lives.

Even so, nothing under the sun could have ever prepared me for the moment when Ali tested positive for a condition so rare that most of the medical community had never heard of it.

At the time, if you Googled "NMO," you would have found little information and even less hope. Most of the content focused on unfortunate accounts of how this disorder could, without warning, bring on blindness, paralysis, and worse. Every parent's darkest nightmare. As if not devastating enough to suddenly find out your beloved child has a life-threatening illness no one can cure—let alone knows much about—it was that much harder to be given the prognosis that our daughter may not live to see her eighteenth birthday.

When my husband and I first heard the doctor speak those words, they were more than shattering. They rearranged the molecules of my mind and soul, ultimately sending me on a mission to lead a cure revolution—even if I didn't know it at the time.

All I knew in those blinding moments was that the Rule of 2% would show me a way forward. How? If 2% had gotten us into this, 2% was going to get us out.

To move toward a solution required me to understand how rare affects everyone.

You might assume, as I once did, that the total number of people afflicted by rare and/or autoimmune illnesses is not very high. Think again.

Dr. Michael Yeaman, a pioneering immunologist and a leading partner in our work to cure NMO—and whose extraordinary vision and voice have guided me on the journey of writing this book—recently put this myth into a global context. Michael has pointed out that the numbers challenge how one defines rare. Given a global population of nearly 7 billion, almost 350 million have a rare disease—and nearly 700 million are estimated to have an autoimmune disease. To give all that perspective, consider this: nearly 10 percent of inhabitants of planet Earth has an autoimmune disease, but only 4 percent uses Twitter. It has been said that if everyone with an autoimmune disease lived in the same land, it would be the third-most-populous country in the world.

No one is immune to disease. Even rare illnesses, taken together, add up to vast numbers of lives impacted and loved ones lost.

Today in the United States alone, more than 30 million people—1 in 10—wake up every morning to the reality of a rare, life-threatening, or debilitating autoimmune condition. There are approximately 7,000 identified rare diseases, almost all of them without cures, and 95 percent have precious few or no treatments.

And to add heartache to misfortune, a high percentage of rare patients are young—with otherwise promising but unlived lives ahead of them. Further, autoimmune diseases are even more unfair, striking women much more frequently than men, and often in the prime of life, during child-bearing years and when children need their mothers more than ever. Such are the tragic and daunting realities of rare and autoimmune diseases.

But there is a new hope emerging—catalyzed by the Power of Rare—and not a moment too soon.

This is the extraordinary story that the NMO community has collectively written. From rare patients to equally rare problem solvers who together take on even rarer challenges, it tells of breakthroughs that have revealed NMO to be the *little disease that could*. Indeed, solving this one rare autoimmune disease could unlock doors to solving all other autoimmune diseases—or beyond, to even more common diseases, including cancer. After all, while such diseases may seem very different on their surface, at their core lies a basic identity crisis in the immune system.

This bold and meaningful understanding about the Power of Rare was echoed recently by filmmaker Jesse Dylan of Wondros films, who has collaborated with us on several short films we created to educate the world about NMO. As Jesse reminded me, this thesis has also been considered in the arena of cancer research.

"What people forget," Jesse said, "is that thirty and forty years ago innovations that came in cancer were from the study of rare cancers. In solving one pathway in one disease, you can then extrapolate it to other pathways. So by focusing like never before on this one condition, NMO, it makes better medicine for everybody."

Medical experts point out similar kinds of breakthroughs. Take for instance the fact that the first medicines to prevent HIV from targeting immune cells were not discovered by studying those who acquired the disease but by studying the rarer individuals who did not, even though they had been exposed.

And NMO takes these concepts further. We know that on the mysterious and miraculous continuum of immune function, too little can make a person vulnerable to cancer or infection, while too much can cause autoimmune disease or worse. Collectively cancer, infection, and autoimmune disease arguably cause more suffering and death than all other conditions combined. By solving NMO, we are learning the secrets of the immune system that control its most basic functions—from why cancer cells or infections elude immunity to why the immune system attacks one's own body in autoimmune disease and everything in between. Imagine the potential these new insights offer for arresting disease at its source—even before it has come to exist at all. That is one Power of Rare.

These realities matter . . . and timing is everything. We are entering a once-in-a-generation window when basic science, clinical medicine, game-changing technology, industry investment, and the Power of Rare are poised together to make quantum leaps in saving and improving lives. In turn, lessons learned and discoveries made by applying the Power of Rare will reveal ideas and resources that can make a world of difference for untold numbers of patients and their loved ones who face rare *and* common diseases.

We need these kinds of solutions more than ever. We are at a crossroads of big challenges and even bigger opportunities. On one hand, we're facing projections of dramatic increases—if not pandemics—of autoimmune disease, as well as cancer and infection. These trends could soon cause unprecedented illness and death around the world—unless we take action *now*. Superbugs are outsmarting antibiotics and threaten to return civilization to the pre-antibiotic era—unless we do something *today*. The climate crisis connected to global warming is sparking new and dangerous rare diseases—in the face of increasing airborne and waterborne threats—and will continue to do so unless we overcome our fears and act *this moment*.

We are all being called to act because the opportunity to solve or even prevent these crises in new and unifying ways has never been so possible.

Never before in the history of human accomplishments have we had the capability to cure NMO and a slew of other rare and even common diseases—thanks to an unprecedented chance to bring together brave new realities: an advanced understanding of the immune system; the technology to address genetic, molecular, and cellular dysfunctions; a global network of industry and advocacy willing to invest in solutions; and a heroic patient community committed to putting their lives on the line.

Yes, I have learned a lot from my against-all-odds journey with a rare disease—and the amazing speed of life advances we have made in just a few short years. How have these advances been achieved? How has this happened? For starters, by redefining rare—by choosing to see and solve the problem differently, and by gathering a group of dedicated problem solvers to join the mission.

This was the case that I presented to the tech gurus in Silicon Valley about why a giant bioinformatics company division should choose to care about a tiny and rare autoimmune disease—for the higher good of making a difference for all.

The truth is that in the universe of rare, people don't always care. If it isn't clear how a disease affects them or their loved ones, most don't connect. Understandable—but unfortunate. And in fairness, it can be hard to see how rare has anything to do with someone not affected by it. This raises another aspect of the work that needs to be done. The reality is that even as the cures of tomorrow require breakthroughs in science and technology today, I believe the concept of a rare disease has a messaging problem—even a marketing problem—that when solved will play a key role in the cure revolution. Caring about rare should matter to us all. And that's one reason that every time I've been disappointed by how people can shrug off the plight of a patient stigmatized by the label of a rare or orphan disease, I've become even more dedicated to telling my "Power of Rare" story in the cause of life-saving solutions.

My blueprint for building a foundation for a cure rests on the bedrock that we can turn rare causes into rare solutions. But to do so we need to care about each other—to realize that although a rare disease may seem to have nothing to do with you, there is a connection yet to be learned, and a solution yet to be found. It starts and ends with heart—and heart is all about connections. Our approach has not been conventional in this respect. For each of the key players on our revolutionary team, it has always been personal—often because of a loved one diagnosed with a life-threatening condition. This fact gave us courage to do things differently, sometimes even radically. My belief from the start was that if it was going to take a revolution to get all the greatest minds together and cure NMO—then by God or the universe or karma—that is what we would do.

I have learned that sometimes too much time is spent trying to tackle the huge or even insurmountable problems, when life-saving clues and solutions are held in the hands of rare all around us. We can be empowered to observe more closely, think more openly, and act more boldly in this cure revolution.

These can truly be the days of miracle and wonder.

We are entering a new era of personalized and precision medicine. In the coming years, we may no longer lump patients together who have the same superficial diagnosis. We will apply the lessons that are so intuitive: that each one of us—each life—truly is unique. Every disease condition will be both infinitely rare and not rare at all. Every patient will have her or his own distinct diagnosis, treatment, and cure. Yet another reason to redefine rare.

The Power of Rare is a book I was inspired to write and that I wrote to inspire. It is a call to action for a constructive revolution to change medicine from one-size-fits-all to custom-tailored care. If I have learned anything in accomplishing many of the things we were told could not easily be done—or be done at all—it is simply that heart and intuition can be as powerful as science and data. Combined, they form a blueprint for achieving the cures that one day can conquer all disease.

Beyond facts and figures, beyond the wonders of technology, we desperately need a revolution in caring—so that we can do this together and that no one is left to bear the burden of rare alone.

Hope is not rare. Love, courage, intuition, and the resiliency to keep going, even in the dark—none of these are rare. Strength in numbers, when the numbers would say otherwise, is rare. And the magical irony is that creating a movement to solve illnesses now considered rare will make them even rarer—to the point that they will become the ultimate example of rare: they will disappear.

After I told them my story of bringing together so many diverse and improbable partners, one of the young execs at Google asked me one simple question. "How? How did you bring all of these competitors together and get them to collaborate?"

It occurred to me that *Saving Each Other*, the book I co-authored with Ali about how we overcame those nightmarish early days following her diagnosis, really spoke to the question of *why* I took on the cause. And now the time had come to write about my blueprint that informed *what* we've done and *how* I have led our team—as we continue to push the boundaries of possibilities for cures at every turn.

My sincere hope is that by my sharing the lessons learned along the way—from the challenges faced to the course corrections made and the victories won—you will be inspired to apply the universal elements of our blueprint to your own revolution for change, whatever the highest goals of your mission may be.

And more, I hope that even in these most promising yet turbulent of times, this book will shed a light on your own miraculous possibilities—that it finds a way into your heart and inspires you to recognize your own uncommon gifts for transforming the world we share for the better.

This is *The Power of Rare*.

THE BLUEPRINT

One has to decide whether one's fears
or one's hopes are
what should matter most.
—Atul Gawande
Being Mortal

CHAPTER 1

OUT OF THE BLUE

A wince. Nothing more.

Out of the blue one night in February 2008—three months shy of her fifteenth birthday—my daughter, Ali, glanced out our car window as the two of us sped off to a mother-daughter night on the town. Then—suddenly she winced.

That moment changed the trajectory of our lives forever. And, because no one is immune, the cascade of events that followed revealed one of the most universal challenges every one of us must face when a nightmare scenario becomes real. It's a matter of survival: the choice to recoil in the face of all-consuming, legitimate fears or to reach for our highest, innate strengths and abilities—and choose hope. And faith.

All of that was foreshadowed in Ali's wince. But that is not where our story begins.

Before that moment, what comes most to mind are memories of a charmed life. By that, I mean in the days and months and years leading up to that point, life for me and my family seemed to be mostly solid, secure, exciting, successful, and somewhat glamorous—in short, charmed.

The charmed life was less about the rarefied air we sometimes inhabited and more about living every day as a blessing to cherish. For me, as a mom, most of all it meant that my three beautiful kids were healthy, happy, and thriving.

As self-made entrepreneurs, my husband, Bill, and I stayed grounded in never forgetting where we came from and in remembering the challenges we had overcome. In our own way, each of us had built a life that reflected what the American Dream is all about—reaching beyond conventional limits, transforming vision into reality. This meant using imagination and innovation to take on the status quo, and having the courage to think and to be different. Beyond our individual successes, we were passionate philanthropists, mentors as well as motivators. Whether paying forward or giving back, I valued opportunities to help create happier, more fruitful lives for others too. But most of all, my charmed life was about family, immediate and extended. About community.

No matter how busy the demands of our businesses, social lives, and other commitments, in our home, family has always come first. Connection has always been the priority.

Each one of my kids has a strong sense of wanting to make a difference in the lives of others and to give back. Even as a little girl, Ali was that way. And not because she wanted to draw attention to herself. Looking back, I'm sure she would have much preferred to go on a quest to end world hunger than put herself out there as Patient Zero for the Power of Rare. But as I would learn, you don't always get to choose the path—often it chooses you.

Once upon a time there was the charmed life with Ali. Then a wince came totally out of the blue one clear Los Angeles night—that would test every meaning of the word "charmed."

THE EYEBALL HEADACHE

Of course it was nothing, I rationalized to myself. But deep down I could feel the shock wave. Call it a sixth sense or mother's intuition.

What had just happened? Minutes before we'd been talking away about the fun we were going to have at the Hollywood premiere of a movie that promised to be a twist on the old Cinderella story. We were, as always, savoring our Mom and Ali time. So much was happening for her—classes and tennis and the school newspaper, to name a few things. A born leader, Ali pulled everything off with grace and peak performance—enough to make the most A-type personality reassess perfection. She managed to inject humor, a sense of adventure, and wisdom beyond her age into every endeavor. She found meaning in every aspect of her bright young life.

After the wince, Ali tried to downplay it, saying, "You know, it feels like an eyeball headache, like something heavy is in my eye." She brushed it off—her way of letting me know there was nothing to worry about. Typical teenager cool. That was pretty much her modus operandi—Ali smooth—no matter what.

Using her daughter logic, Ali would be the first to say that she did not have to worry about anything like an eyeball headache because: a) she knew for certain that whatever the problem was, she could count on Mom to fix it; and b) why sweat it when Mom does all the worrying for everyone else?

True. I decided long ago that shielding my three beloved kids from worry was part of my job as Mom—*right?*

Until early 2008, my *career* job was leading the cosmetics company I had launched twenty years earlier from my garage—and that I built into a global brand. But my profession never defined me. My identity has always been much more rooted in being a mother.

Ironically, instead of listening to my darker voice of concern about Ali's sudden blurred vision and eye pain, for once I convinced myself all would be fine after we got her the right prescription for eye drops or whatever the doctor ordered. After all, we were talking about an otherwise healthy teenager.

"Optic neuritis." That was the official diagnosis made by the eye doctor. Although I had never heard the term before, it seemed simple

enough—a little bit of "eye-itis" did not seem to be a life-or-death problem. I thought we could take care of this minor issue and move on. But
before I could exhale, the doctor referred Ali to a neurologist colleague
for further testing. My "mom alarm" was now reverberating concern as the
first shoe dropped.

"Why?" My stomach knotted up.

He had already prescribed steroids that he assured me would soon
reduce the swelling and probably clear up her blurred eyesight quickly
and permanently.

"Because," he explained, "it's important to find out *why* she is having
the optic nerve inflammation in the first place."

Today, I am grateful for that doctor's hunch that maybe there was
something more going on. I now realize we were fortunate, as many patients are only treated for symptoms—with little investigation as to their
cause. But at the time I was unnerved: if the steroids would clear up the
condition, then why more tests? That was my "mom heart" trying to spare
Ali concern. Even so, my "mom mind" made the appointment with the
specialist and agreed to additional blood work.

That's when the other shoe dropped. I watched this kindly and thor-
ough neurologist checking off boxes on a laboratory form that listed
possible blood tests he could order for Ali to rule out a whole host of potential causes for her eyeball headache. Normally, I would not have even
looked at the test names or asked questions. What did I know, anyway?
But there was something eerie about one test he ordered that included in
fine print the letters "NMO-IgG."

Whatever prompted me to say anything, I have no idea, but not missing a beat, I asked, "What's that?"

The doctor reassured me it was only to rule out something very rare
and entirely unlikely. "Don't worry," he said. "She won't have that." He
then mumbled something about how that would be too terrible to contemplate—a nightmare.

NMO—a simple three-letter abbreviation for a very complex disease
known as neuromyelitis optica. The condition was so rare—I would later

learn—that he had never heard any colleague report the test coming back positive, much less ever encountered a patient who had it. As the test was new and had only been developed a few years earlier at the Mayo Clinic, this was the first time he had ever tested anyone for the nightmare.

AGAINST ALL ODDS

What happened next blurred time and space in a collision of anguish in my memory. It's hard to recall how many days lapsed before Bill and I huddled over the phone in our home office and waited to hear a report from the additional tests. There were so many results to review, I told myself worrying was useless. Surely there would be a common diagnosis with an easy fix.

But during those next surreal seconds, that assumption was destroyed. We were told Ali had tested positive for a condition that was among the rarest of the rare. I vaguely remember first hearing the terms "neuromyelitis optica" and NMO for short—as if the simple name would mean a simple treatment.

Previously known as Devic's disease, NMO is anything but simple. As we would learn, this rare autoimmune disease of the central nervous system involves two of the most complex and mysterious aspects of the human body—the brain and the immune system. We were then given what little information the neurologist knew about NMO—and were told to prepare ourselves for the worst.

There *had* to be a mistake. Someone or some test must be incorrect. I stopped breathing.

There is no book, no guide, no platitudes or proverbs that can prepare anyone to grapple with news of a rare diagnosis and horrifying prognosis for their dearest loved ones. You feel plunged into darkness, without even a crack of light to be found. A charmed world of color and laughter turned gray and silent. We felt utterly alone—and Ali's life was on the line.

In one instant, my story changed from having overcome all odds to being up against all odds.

INTO A SEA OF DARKNESS

In 2008, there was precious little information available about NMO and none easily accessed online—except for a few gothic accounts of how this mysterious disorder could strike without warning and wreak devastating havoc. It was so rare that the majority of healthcare providers had never heard of NMO, much less seen a case in real life.

It should be enough of a terrifying specter to suddenly learn that your beloved child has what experts call an "incurable" and life-threatening condition that few know about. But even more than that, we were now on watch for the sudden and mysterious onset of another attack that would mean the advancement of the disease. This is one of the most brutal fears a mother can have—that NMO relapses can occur without warning or mercy, and that their cumulative effects can leave a loved one blind and paralyzed—as if cast adrift into a sea of darkness.

The menace of NMO onset or relapse can be accompanied by a host of symptoms: terrible pain, inability to control bowel or bladder function, loss of eyesight, inability to move, and sometimes a range of peculiar gastrointestinal issues such as uncontrollable hiccups. But even the lightning bolt shock of such scenarios paled in comparison to what I remember hearing on that same phone call: "This would be the time to try to make the most of however long you have left with your daughter." We had been told to prepare for loss.

From that moment, I began to hear the sound of a ticking clock in my head. Call it a ticking time bomb.

In the days that followed, we confronted other realities about this rare and poorly understood disease that had no treatments proven to be effective or safe, and even less hope of breakthrough research.

However much I wanted to fall apart and rage against the universe, that would have to wait and could not be my ultimate choice. The truth is that no disease, regardless how rare or relentless, could curse my capacity to respond. Nor could it shatter the deepest part of my heart, from where I would draw the power to defy the odds. As little as I knew about NMO, nothing could conquer my resolve that there was no such thing as "impossible" when it came to our bold intention: saving Ali and ensuring she would not just survive but thrive and live a long, healthy life filled with joy.

I had so much to learn. The physical lessons of science and medicine would be a must. But the metaphysical lesson of the eyeball headache came first—that no matter how happy, secure, or charmed a life may seem, no one is guaranteed protection from a terrifying diagnosis. And while each human life is singular in its own way, none of us gets a pass from the necessity to act in the face of our fears. The "worst" was not going to happen—not on my watch.

A CENTURY OF MYSTERY

Looking back, there was shockingly little information about NMO readily available to the newly diagnosed. To this injury, add the insult that NMO was labeled an "orphan" disease—meaning it was assigned a classification that in a numbers game could stand in the way of funding for promising research or new drug trials.

As an outsider to how slow-moving medical research can be, it was natural to be all the more alarmed that this mysterious rare disease had fallen through the cracks of medical science. But that wasn't the ultimate surprise. The greater surprise was how the Power of Rare—what I would soon recognize as a source to give us answers—had been so long neglected in NMO or other exceptionally uncommon diseases. A different way of thinking about rare was desperately needed to galvanize the science of a disease that was mostly mired in the quicksand of nineteenth-century dogma.

In time, I would catch up on the history of how this condition had remained in the dark for the last century. Then I had to cobble together this background into a mosaic of opportunity—enough to eventually let me glimpse how solving NMO could unlock the mystery of other unsolved diseases.

Neuro-myélite optique aigue—or neuromyelitis optica acuta—was the name given this elusive disease in 1894 by a young French neurologist named Eugène Devic and his medical student Fernand Gault. It was first described as a syndrome of the central nervous system, in which many of Devic's patients presented with acute symptoms resembling multiple sclerosis. A condition of rapid onset in which both the spinal cord and optic nerves were affected, it was known to afflict more women than men. The disorder had mystified early researchers for its refusal to follow any kind of predictable course. Infections such as botulism, heritable blindness, spinal cord trauma, or even obscure mental illnesses were among the initial considerations as causes. It was a true orphan condition that had never been systematically studied or appropriated to any single branch of medical research. So, for lack of any other parent, Devic adopted the condition he had first called neuromyelitis optica as his own to study, and, as suggested by Gault, Devic's disease became the name of the syndrome.

Then, for more than a hundred years, the science and medical practice of NMO remained a mystery. Small advances, derived from passing glimpses into the effects of NMO, occurred from time to time—whenever an impassioned doctor tried to push the boundaries of medical care to change the devastating course of disease. But even the most modern therapies of those periods were not yet proven safe or effective, and posed their own concerns associated with a lengthy suppression of the immune system.

Devic's disease continued for the most part to be considered an extreme, highly aggressive variant of multiple sclerosis (MS) until a breakthrough was reported in December 2004 from the Mayo Clinic:

ROCHESTER, MN—Misdiagnosis of a severely paralyzing disease can now be averted due to a blood test developed by Mayo Clinic researchers and their Japanese collaborators. Often misdiagnosed as multiple sclerosis, neuromyelitis optica (NMO) also causes blindness in many sufferers. The finding will help doctors correctly treat NMO—also known as Devic's syndrome—sooner and more effectively. Early diagnosis is important because NMO is best treated differently than multiple sclerosis. Treatment requires immune suppressive medications in the first instance, rather than the immune modulatory treatments typically prescribed for MS. Therefore, a patient who has NMO, but is misdiagnosed with MS, may not receive optimal care at the earliest possible time.

The news described how their scientific investigation had led to the discovery of a characteristic autoantibody—an immune system protein that circulated in the bloodstream and targeted the normally harmless water channel molecule, aquaporin-4 (AQP4). At first, because this anti-body was identified in just a small subset of 85,000 blood samples taken from patients with different autoimmune disorders, its significance was not understood. But when the sample codes were broken, the researchers discovered that the mystery autoantibody was present only in the blood of NMO patients. From that day forward, the telltale autoantibody was given the name NMO-immunoglobulin G—or NMO-IgG—and served as a biomarker to help diagnose this rare autoimmune disease.

Unfortunately, key discoveries take time to be accepted—even in the life-and-death arena of medicine. Although the NMO-IgG biomarker was known, even the U.S. National Institutes of Health (NIH) had few answers for causes or consequences of NMO as late as 2007. Their NMO "fact sheet" offered as few facts as the cases they attempted to describe:

NMO leads to loss of myelin, which is a fatty substance that surrounds nerve fibers and helps nerve signals move from cell to cell. The syndrome can also damage nerve fibers and leave areas of broken-down tissue. In the disease process of NMO, for reasons that aren't yet clear, immune system cells and antibodies attack and destroy myelin cells in the optic nerves and the spinal cord.

And worse, hardly any of the information that was known about NMO was available to newly diagnosed patients or their loved ones. No organized mechanism was in place to raise awareness of—or access to—the blood test for NMO-IgG. So countless patients continued to be misdiagnosed with MS or other conditions and, in many cases, were administered medicines that did not help them or even harmed them. None of this was the fault of clinicians, NIH, or any other entity. NMO was simply too rare a disease for physicians to know otherwise, or to rise high enough on their radar screen of urgency. Those barriers would be shattered at the speed of life, as we would describe the pace of change that had to happen beginning in 2008.

JOURNEY TO THE LAND OF MAYO

When Bill and I hung up from that nightmarish call, our world plunged into darkness. We sat in frozen silence for moments, staring at the phone—as if it was to blame for the horrifying news we had just received. A wrong number? Somebody else's curse? The doctor had actually said to us, "This would be the time to go into denial."

Somewhere in that blur, wracked with anguish and disbelief, I could barely feel my body as I made it up the stairs to our bedroom, where I broke down. My next thoughts—when I could start to form them, after peeling myself off the floor—started coming in a flood of urgent questions. *How can I protect my daughter? What must I learn about this rare autoimmune condition? Where are the experts who know more? Who is leading the charge for research? When will there be promising treatments and a cure? Are there other patients and families we can talk to? Or are we alone?*

We immediately began scouring every possible source of information there was to be found about this "incurable orphan disease"—from the Internet to medical literature and beyond. We quickly sought out all expertise in our own medical Rolodex, and extended it into a six-degrees-of-connection network. The consensus from every link was to get ourselves to the Mayo Clinic in Rochester, Minnesota. As in—*get there yesterday.*

That March, we flew from balmy, tropical Los Angeles into the late winter weather of the Land of 10,000 Lakes. In the midst of Minnesota snow flurries, with most of our family seated in the waiting room, courage and fear came closest together.

Everything was locked in time, still and quiet. In my memory we were surrounded by darkness, with only our faces lit, as in a Rembrandt portrait, foretelling a story of shadows and hopes that no words could express. Ali appeared to me as though draped in the white light I had been summoning to protect her. Calm. Stoic.

Even with my best intentions, she had not failed to notice the signs—Center for Multiple Sclerosis and Autoimmune Neurology and Neuro-immunology and Demyelinating Diseases.

"Do I have MS?" Ali asked. Just a day earlier she was content to leave the answer to her questions at "too much inflammation." In fact, she had explicitly asked not to know more about her diagnosis. I told her, "No, honey, that's not what you have." She nodded and reverted back to that cryptic glint in her eyes. The one that says, 'Nuff' said. That's all I need to know—for now.

No words were needed to remind me that I was supposed to fix this. This is what I do. And that was all Ali wanted to know.

But her face registered a pulse of concern—a tiny vein that showed itself on her brow. It was the same endearing little blue sign of life she had as a newborn that seemed extraordinary, even rare. It was the kind of sign that made me think one day things might not go so easily for this little angel. And then all at once time and space snapped me back to the reality that I knew she was thinking: Why? Why am I here?

Yes, why were we here? After all, since the "eyeball headache," Ali's optic neuritis had improved. The steroids had done their job. After watching her vision in the one eye diminish to the point that she could no longer tell how many fingers I was holding up in front of her nose, her eyesight had almost returned to normal. But there we were, in the Mayo Clinic waiting room, anticipating our meeting with Dr. Brian Weinshenker.

With its mystique for offering solutions after long and difficult personal journeys, the Mayo Clinic represented a metaphor for the Land of Oz—the magical place out of one of Ali's favorite stories. Dr. Weinshenker was the expert we had traveled to see, and the man we would come to respectfully call the "Wizard of Mayo."

I noticed Ali taking in the room, assessing the other patients also waiting to be seen. Some were sight-impaired. Some were paralyzed, in wheelchairs, or only able to walk with the aid of canes, walkers, or loved ones. They were young and old, but none as young as Ali. Their family members and caretakers showed a spectrum of emotion from concern to hope—from exhaustion to fear.

The difference between them and us, I sensed, was that none appeared to be newly diagnosed. None of them had that air of denial you expect to see on the faces of people who have not spent much time in waiting rooms—the ones whose body language and expressions suggest, *Don't mind us . . . we're just passing through.*

But what if we were not just passing through? This dread-filled question reared up over and over.

Is this where we are going to live now?

No, I told myself. *This isn't us.*

But I knew better. My intuition was already in overdrive, warning me not to believe this would be an easy walk on a temporary road. Even while trying to argue the diagnosis away, I was feeling a crisis of compass—disorienting all my reference points, all my defenses. In this fearful blur, I vividly recall the concern on Dr. Weinshenker's face after examining Ali and running more tests. We sent her to the lobby to play cards with her grandmother, and he ushered us into his office.

In the land of life-threatening and poorly understood diseases—a labyrinth with no seeming escape—the bespectacled, visionary Dr. Weinshenker shone with apparent magical powers to guide us to a better place. With the gravity of a clinical wizard, he was youngish in appearance—but ageless in wisdom. Had he raised a wand to make all concerns about Ali vanish, I would have believed him. Instead, with a kind blend of compassion and reality that only comes from years of conveying difficult truths, and with an expression of absolute certainty, he confirmed, "Textbook NMO."

He explained, "The pattern for many patients is that the optic nerve is the first to come under attack." He predicted it would probably be just a matter of months before the next phase: the transverse myelitis or spinal cord attacks. Tingling, numbness, pain, paralysis.

In panic-driven, breathless desperation, I asked, "Couldn't this be a one-time thing?" I mentioned again that her eyesight was almost back completely and there had only been the one attack. "Could we not be seeing something so rare," I asked, "a milder or even benign version of the condition that has never been seen before? Would it be possible that we're going to skip the transverse myelitis?"

As much as we could all hope for that possibility, Dr. Weinshenker said it was not likely.

And in textbook fashion, Ali would in fact suffer her first spinal attack a few months later.

Even though we were hoping against hope he would be wrong, we didn't wait to take action for Ali. He advised us to immediately begin an aggressive approach to treatment. A combined regimen of powerful immune suppressants and drugs normally used to treat cancers.

Few hopes—fewer options.

Welcome to the catch-22 for so many autoimmune disease patients. By suppressing the immune system, one goal is to mute the identity crisis that results in the immune system attacking the very body it was designed to protect. But in doing so, such treatments also limit the immune system from fending off equally dangerous threats of infection, cancer—or worse. For these patients, even the commonest of colds could become life-threatening.

The sobering news Dr. Weinshenker delivered next was that there were no surefire treatments for NMO—and no guarantees. Each patient was different—rare unto themselves—when it came to which medicines, and which cocktail of combinations of those medicines, *might* be effective. But no regimen would be without side effects.

By this point, I had already learned about the barriers to research for rare orphan diseases and, generally, why drugs to effectively treat these conditions were so few and far between. Yet the impact of these limitations never hit home until that moment. What came to me was a bare-bones concept that appeared almost as unexpectedly as Ali's diagnosis. At that moment, between despair and hope, our foundation was conceived.

It was much more than simply a conscious decision. It was a mother's sheer resolve—as the words began to fall out of me. I heard myself say to

Dr. Weinshenker, "You don't know me, but I have a checkbook, and we're going to be getting to know each other very well."

REVOLUTION FROM WITHIN

At the instant of its origin, I could not have fully envisioned that we were starting a world-class foundation that would bend time and space to discover new treatments and cures for NMO. Nor could I have predicted that I would become a colleague on a global team of the best and brightest minds from across the medical and scientific spectrum. All I knew was that we were up against unacceptable odds, that we had to find our power to change them, and that we needed to act quickly and wisely.

If courage is the best friend of optimism, fear is the companion of reality. I had no grand vision for how this would play out. Neither did I have any real idea of the challenges facing anyone with a rare orphan autoimmune disease. What's more, I had yet to fathom the scourge of autoimmune conditions that were already rising to epidemic levels. What I did know was that by starting with science we would lay the stepping-stones to safe and effective treatments—and ultimately a cure—for NMO and beyond.

By June 2008, after Ali suffered her first transverse myelitis attack, the framework for the Guthy-Jackson Charitable Foundation (GJCF) was already in place, but there was no blueprint. There was no realization that a medical revolution was stirring. Not yet.

For that to happen, a personal revolution had to take place—the kind that Gloria Steinem calls *the revolution from within*. My story would be that of any mom—or Everymom—or anyone who chooses hope over fear for a struggle they've never undertaken before. And, for lack of a better phrase, becomes the change they want to see in the world. Faith told me there was an organic way forward for a personal revolution that had already begun from within. There was a pathway with lessons not at all rare but universal—to be applied by me or by anyone who faces a challenge others would call insurmountable.

Those lessons are among the profound truths I have learned since Ali was first struck by a rare diagnosis, and they have helped me find the strength and resilience to go on:

- No life is immune to being shattered without warning— whether by a terrifying mystery diagnosis or an unforeseen tragedy. Yet the same truth that says we cannot always see into the future also says we have the power to choose how to face it and change it.
- Denial is always an option—but it's never a good one. As much as we wish the problem never happened, the reality is what it is. And that's where revolution begins.
- The gift of choice is a power that all too often we forget. We can choose to be alone and isolated in the solitude of rare—or we can choose to accept rare as a powerful fuel to give voice and heart and value to each life.
- The difference between hope and fear is not one of black and white. Not a day goes by that I don't feel fearful. But not a day goes by that I don't wake up asking myself what I can learn, do, or change to let hope determine the future.
- When you find yourself in a sea of darkness and there seems nothing you can do—choose to do something, anything, not to sink. When there is no wind, row.
- Reality is that uncomfortable but necessary stretch of land that exists between impossible and possible. Learn from it, gain clarity from it, and use reality to begin your revolution from within.

My focus from the start was on putting one foot in front of the other and building our organization in record time to find answers and save lives—beginning with our daughter's.

To do that, I needed to believe it *could* be done. Then I needed to learn how it *would* be done.

The future depends entirely on what each of us does every day.

—Gloria Steinem

CHAPTER 2

MOM ON A MISSION

You never truly know the depths of your innermost strengths or the limitlessness of your rare powers until you are called to action for a cause that is your own do-or-die—when *do* is the only acceptable outcome.

When there is no user's blueprint, it's only natural to wonder how on earth you begin. One answer that has been a mainstay for me is that you start where you are. Create your own plan—use everything you know and everything you are. To do that, as the saying goes, you must first "know thyself."

Knowing ourselves means we must be both harsh critics and gentle counselors—so that we can know our limits as well as our strengths. Being honest and accepting of both can make it easier to confront the status quo. And, as I would soon learn, knowing thyself also happens to be an essential metaphor for understanding and unraveling a rare autoimmune disease.

TRUSTING YOUR INSTINCTS

When I made the decision to lead the charge in taking on NMO, I immediately heard many of the same criticisms I learned to disregard as a cosmetics entrepreneur who had challenged the old-school dogma of the beauty world. When I was building my business and putting it on the map, I did my best to ignore comments like: "That's not how it's done" and "It'll never work" and "You don't have the expertise."

I was told my unconventional approach to "no makeup makeup" would never succeed. But it did—and wildly. Investors predicted failure when I pitched the idea of selling color cosmetics via an infomercial format that I intended to elevate with high-quality production values and personal, relatable storytelling. They were wrong.

The lesson from those chapters of my life was a powerful one—to trust my instincts and not to sell myself short. This lesson is at the heart of the Power of Rare: learn to trust and leverage that which sets you apart, no matter the pushback.

For as much as I didn't know yet, there was no way I could outsource this job to someone else—no matter how capable or how knowledgeable. Once you choose to turn over that leadership role, the mission is no longer in your control, and you have lost your power. Of course, I knew we would need to build a world-class team to join the effort of battling NMO, and work with them rather than watch from the sideline. Still, whatever our strides were to be, those were on me to help inspire.

Yes, there were moments when I could have fantasized about a real-life Wizard of Oz to find the cure or someone who could wave a magic wand and make NMO disappear. Yet as a realist, I have always known that the "person behind the curtain" is really *you*.

It's true. There are no wand wavers or all-powerful wizards who can make the magic for you. You have to lead.

I was Ali's mom, and I chose to accept that the universe, fairly or unfairly, had assigned me the job of solving NMO. No one was going to care as much or be as motivated as me. To gather the right people and inspire them to invest their time and expertise in our cause, I felt they would first need to see that I was for real—and involved in every aspect of the operation.

Even if I hadn't done anything like this before, for us all to succeed, I'd need to trust in myself that I could do this.

Did I know we were going to be the only ones on the job of solving NMO at the time? Not exactly.

At the very beginning, I imagined our foundation could focus on funding research that was already under way, or perhaps join forces with others actively working on NMO. We studied, we asked, we Googled. It quickly became clear we were the only game in town. Still, the prospect of charting our own course and cutting through the proverbial red tape would ultimately be liberating.

But none of that gave us any comfort in those summer months of 2008 that followed Ali's first transverse myelitis attack. In the all-encompassing center of uncertainty and fear that comes with a cruel diagnosis of a beloved child, there are few truths that will hold fast. From the moment we had first heard of NMO, we had been told to focus on the worst—to prepare for sorrow.

Every minute tore me in two directions—whether to hold Ali in my arms or let her go to experience all she could in whatever time remained. I needed to do both and then defy the odds too.

Somewhere in that frozen state of being, I summoned the survival lessons that were in my DNA and in my own life journey—from a premature birth I shouldn't have survived and the first months of life spent in the hospital to prolonged childhood illnesses and an unstable home life to learning how to make my own way in the working world from the time I was a teenager. Those survival instincts that visited me in the dark were welcome reminders of my resilience. If those capacities were in my wiring, wouldn't they be in Ali's too? Of course they were.

The necessity to solve NMO had forever altered my identity and made my purpose clear. If there was no one else spearheading the job of stopping this rare autoimmune killer, it would be—it could only be—me.

There would be no opting out.

A RARE APPROACH TO A RARE DISEASE

The Latin term "de novo" means to arise from nothing. What we were up against called for a de novo blueprint for the work of the Foundation. Conventional models of medical philanthropy followed old-school rules: bring in management experts and let them run the show. Progress, if it occurred, would be slow. Our blueprint would be different. We had to steer this mothership at a much faster pace than the traditional rules allowed.

Once again, I dismissed the naysayers who argued that was not how it was done and that I had never taken on a challenge like this. I knew better.

When facing a life-or-loss situation, I believe a transformation takes place deep inside you—at a molecular level. I had to run every aspect of this operation differently. In that pressure cooker, focus was fundamental.

When you finally accept—*"Oh, my God, this is happening . . ."*—you have to come up with a way to change the future, and *now*; and I had to get it right.

I chose to develop a rare approach to a rare disease. I chose to create a blueprint that dared to challenge medical dogma. Too often the medical community becomes complacent with familiarity. NMO had been "too complex" or "too rare" or "too *whatever*" to ever have a solution. The time had come for a new era of NMO. Of course, there would be pushback—and more naysayers than ever. But if there were not, then I'd know we weren't really changing anything for the better.

To find the best answers, we needed to ask the best questions. As a visual thinker, it seemed to me that we had to begin by challenging everything that was known about NMO, then reassemble the puzzle in a way that produced a new image—a picture of cures. If my mission was to ultimately unravel the mystery that no one else had, I had to start by learning two foreign languages: immunology and rare disease.

ALL ROADS LEAD TO THE IMMUNE SYSTEM

Over and over, I delved into medical literature for answers from experts who could help educate me about the basic science and medicine of NMO. The deeper I looked, the more I learned that the wonders, complexities, and contradictions of the immune system are at the heart of so many medical issues.

In an early conversation with Dr. Yeaman, I remember him pointing out that cancers, infections, and autoimmune diseases are among the greatest threats to personal and global health. "On their surface," he explained, "these conditions may not seem to have anything in common. Yet at their origins, each of their roads leads to the immune system. The same is true for many medical concerns, from multiple sclerosis to transplant rejection, type 1 diabetes, and wound healing. Likely even aging itself."

Cancers are caused by cells gone rogue. These cells ignore healthy signals telling them when and where to stop growing, and how to do so peacefully. Instead, they grow out of control and, worse, they fool the immune system into seeing them as normal until it is too late. Failure of the immune system to identify and clear rogue cells before they cause disease is at the root of all cancers. So the "cure" for cancer is never to let it get past the sentinels of the immune system in the first place. Finding ways to correct or educate the immune system in advance to seek and destroy cancer cells is key to conquering cancer.

Globally, infection is a leading cause of sickness and death, and the growing threat of antibiotic resistance looms larger every day. Infection results from one of two basic challenges: pathogens that outsmart an immune system or an immune system that is incapable of clearing them. When difficult infections occur, antibiotics are thrown at them, but pathogens can outsmart antibiotics. That's scary enough. I also learned that even the most powerful antibiotic cannot clear infection in the absence of a capable immune system. These facts create a paradox in modern medicine: without effective antibiotics, of course there will be lives harmed and lost due to infection, but beyond that, many modern advances of medicine will simply fade away—from cancer therapy to organ transplantation; from life-sparing surgery to treating autoimmune diseases. The field needed new ideas and new actions. Now.

That brings me to the less obvious but no less ominous and silent creep of autoimmune diseases. I was shocked to discover that, as a group, autoimmune diseases affect two times more patients than do cancers, and as many patients as does heart disease. In contrast to cancer or infection, autoimmune diseases occur when the immune system mistakes molecules, cells, or tissues of the very body it was intended to protect as if they were infection or cancer—and goes on the attack.

What can this mean? Cancer or infection results from too weak an immune response—while autoimmune diseases result from too strong a response . . . . Or a misdirected response. As just one example, Dr. Yeaman noted that recent studies suggest one in five cancers is caused by a preventable infection. If so, millions of cancers can be prevented by educating the immune system in advance to defend against cancer-causing infection. This understanding points to one of the most promising new areas of cancer treatment: immunotherapy. Here, therapeutic antibodies are used to release the brakes of the immune system, so it no longer ignores the cancer cells but chases them down and kills them.

Sounds great . . . right? Well, not so fast. A more complex reality is that one serious side effect of such immunotherapy is autoimmune disease. As with many things in life, balance is everything: too much immune activity is bad, and too little is bad. But as Dr. Yeaman explained, "This 'Goldilocks' effect suggests there is a hidden secret, a master switch of the immune system. If so, mastering the immune system could mean cures for solving some of the greatest disease scourges of humanity."

Wow. Maybe NMO offered the chance to decode rare and special properties of the immune system that could help reveal the secrets of its master switch.

Just to be real, I hadn't forgotten that NMO resides at the rarest of all intersections in the human body—the central nervous system and the immune system. If we were going to conquer this disease, we would have to find answers that would most likely come in the form of rare molecules and cells in already rare patients.

And as if this wasn't complicated enough, add to the NMO equation the fact that the ability of the immune system to know the difference between "self" (e.g., normal healthy tissue) and "nonself" (e.g., foreign microbe or abnormal cancer cell) is fundamental to health. The very same immune functions that cause the immune system to attack its own body in autoimmune diseases are immobilized by cancer cells—killers that should otherwise be sought and destroyed by effective immune identity.

Know thyself, I thought. Then I realized the identity crisis in NMO and other autoimmune diseases offered a powerful and universal message. In the world of beauty, authentic identity is based less on how the world sees us and more on how we see ourselves, and therein lies a parallel to immune health.

If part of our life's journey is to know ourselves—through exploration, contemplation, and action—wouldn't the metaphor of immune identity suggest a road to a cure that could be reached through those same means in medical research?

Though I certainly had no answers, it made sense to me early on that within this most challenging science was the potential for revolutionizing medicine. We were at the threshold of something big. I could see that solving NMO could lead to a better understanding of the basic recognition and response functions of the immune system. So it followed that these same discoveries could then be applied to understanding why the immune system fails to prevent cancer and infection—but is vigilant to a fault when it comes to autoimmune diseases like NMO.

Suddenly, NMO was more than just an obscure disease, and our mission to solve it transcended rare.

THE SILENT EPIDEMIC OF AUTOIMMUNITY

My crash course in immunology and autoimmune disease continued late into every night. As I was getting up to speed on autoimmunity, I found it ironic how little education is provided to the general public about the range and threat of autoimmune diseases. It is true that out of the more than eighty known chronic and debilitating autoimmune diseases, some are rare. But not all. Take type 1 diabetes, for example—believed to affect up to 2 million Americans. And there's Hashimoto's thyroiditis, which afflicts as many as 1 million people in the US alone. Add nearly 1.5 million lupus patients and 2 million rheumatoid arthritis patients to the list in the US, along with collective millions of patients suffering from psoriasis, Crohn's disease, and on and on.

Then there's the population of patients facing multiple sclerosis (MS)—half a million or more in the US and millions more worldwide. This fact may be especially surprising when you consider that MS may be one of the most familiar of all autoimmune diseases—and billions of dollars have been spent trying to understand and cure MS over the years. Even so, to date, MS remains largely a mystery, with no definitive blood biomarker of disease and no way to predict who will be stricken. And while several drugs have been approved to somewhat delay or lessen the severity of relapses in mild forms of MS, there is still no treatment proven effective for its more virulent form—secondary progressive MS—and no cure for any form of the disease. *Unacceptable.*

It was staggering to learn the impact autoimmune diseases have on humankind. The numbers are worth repeating—there are an estimated 30 million US patients directly affected by an autoimmune disease and globally as many as 700 million. The costs of medicines, healthcare, lost wages, and more mean tens of billions of dollars lost each year in the US alone. Add more zeros worldwide, and the cost of rare autoimmune diseases rivals that of any medical priority—from mental health to public health.

Next time you are out at a large party or concert or sporting event, look around—many in the crowd are quietly suffering from the silent epidemic of autoimmune disease. More and more, someone you know or someone connected to you is, or is going to be, directly affected.

To reiterate: Autoimmune diseases mainly target women. In this country, they're already a leading cause of death of women younger than sixty-five. Adding heartache to misfortune, onset of an autoimmune condition often arrives during a woman's child-bearing years. In this context, I learned something else that was both amazing and devastating. Somehow, the same system of immune tolerance—which allows a pregnant mother to carry a fetus that might otherwise be viewed as a foreign object—is turned against her in autoimmune diseases.

Autoimmune diseases limit independence and happiness due to countless medical appointments and always being on guard to avoid infection. Some autoimmune diseases come with disfiguring skin conditions, incontinence, even cognitive problems. For the rare, life-threatening autoimmune diseases such as NMO, burdens are taken to yet another level—blindness, paralysis, or worse. And many of these diseases impose more subtle yet chronic symptoms due to the fact that having one autoimmune disease can increase the chances of getting another one.

The silence was deafening when it came to public awareness of all these concerns. It even seemed the medical community at large was either not paying attention or was just shaking its proverbial head at the oncoming epidemic. Where was the outrage? Where was the global warning system to get ahead of this threat? It was time to make some noise.

A CANARY IN THE COAL MINE

I filled stacks of notebooks with questions and observations from all that I had read and heard. There was one word that cropped up in my notes more than any other. It glared back at me from the pages: *Why?*

Why did NMO emerge at all, or become triggered in patients when there was no clear cause? *Why*, at the time, had no known connections been studied in terms of genetics, environment, or exposure to viruses or infections? What was it that connected the few other NMO patients I had met by the summer of 2008 to Ali? Was it just random?

Then I stumbled upon a description of autoimmune disease as being the modern-day example of a "canary in a coal mine." In the old days, miners would take canaries down into the coalmines with them because the birds were much more sensitive than humans to toxic levels of gases such as carbon monoxide and methane. If the canaries started to become distressed or sick or worse, that alerted the miners that they were in danger and it was time to get out immediately.

Maybe NMO was a canary asking us to look more closely at causes—what experts would later suggest might be an indicator of genes-meet-environment issues in which the immune system suffers an identity crisis. In this light, NMO could be a model of all autoimmune diseases—or, for that matter, all immune dysfunctions in which determining self from nonself was at stake. If so, then it stood to reason that NMO belonged to everyone. Then solving NMO should be everyone's priority.

That would connect us all to the Power of Rare.

SOLVING THE UNSOLVABLE

Even at the beginning of my NMO medical education, I could see the reasons that there would be tremendous momentum to solve NMO if we could show how it connected to solving other diseases—even if the connections were not obvious.

In the fall of 2008, none of the far-reaching benefits of solving NMO were yet part of the conversation. No, our focus was on NMO itself—24/7—and it was encouraging when some of the leading lights in science and medicine began joining our cause.

By this time, I had learned a lot of the medical lingo and could navigate the literature. From the difference between T cells and B cells to the difference between downstream effects and upstream causes—it made sense. And this knowledge placed on the table a universe of possibilities for research and development that might help find cures. But it's worth repeating that there's a big difference between what *could* be done and what *should* be done. For my team—for the sake of Ali and all NMO patients—every action taken or not taken had to be mission-critical.

I wanted immediate, tangible, and real help for Ali. From the start, I absolutely believed that sitting on some shelf or in a test tube archive in the basement of some drug company was a better treatment for NMO sufferers than the options available. And it turned out that this vision was not entirely at odds with the medical establishment. As I later learned, this was the concept of *repurposing*—redirecting a drug originally discovered or applied for one disease and using it to benefit patients suffering from another. Even so, we needed to move more quickly than the snail's pace of twelve to fifteen years or more that it usually took to get new drugs into clinical trials.

But my main departure from the beaten path was in declaring my belief that this was not just a mission to delay or treat NMO—but to *cure* it. Even using that word was simply not done. We were told it was too bold, too hopeful.

Yet all the lessons of my life pointed to one truth that helped to shape our mission. It was at the same time simple and profound. One of the great barriers to solving the unsolvable is thinking there can be no solution. I focused on the alternative: *What if? Why not?—Say yes.* My intuition reminded me that miracles are only granted to those who believe they are possible.

That is when I understood the need for a true medical revolution. Not a destructive exercise in blame—or churning up chaos and calamity—but a positive pathway to collaborations and cures. If, as we were out to prove, NMO had a cause that was definable and targetable for treatment to stop it, why not go forward with the highest intention to move beyond halting the disease to reversing it? Not only did I want to believe and visualize these possibilities and have them motivate me, but our fledgling foundation agreed to go against the status quo and declare as our mission mantra: "The Guthy-Jackson Charitable Foundation is dedicated to funding research in the quest to understand Neuromyelitis Optica (NMO) Spectrum Disorder . . . is passionate in its support of programs and opportunities aimed at changing the clinical paradigm for NMO patients . . . and is undaunted in its effort to improve treatment, enable prevention and find *an eventual cure for this disease.*"

Of course, saying this was the easy part. Making it happen would be another story. Machinery for a cure had to be built—and most of its parts didn't even exist yet.

A ROSE BY ANY OTHER NAME

In the world of makeup, I eagerly borrowed from older models and successes while always looking for ways to be new and original. And though building a medical foundation was entirely different from perfecting my cosmetics foundation, many of the same principles applied to both. For our new blueprint, we combined tradition with innovation and life-and-death urgency to overcome obstacles in ways that had never been done before.

But I was not the one who truly breathed life into our new-school foundation. No—that inspiration came from Ali herself. During the several months that followed her official diagnosis, Ali had yet to ask or want to know the actual name of her condition. Even as she navigated the painful and unpredictable attacks of NMO, it was always with grace and resilience. She rarely complained about the vein-piercing treatments, appetite-ruining pills, claustrophobic MRI scans, or countless medical appointments. She learned the many ways that NMO makes itself a most unwelcome visitor in the lives of those who have it. Yet Ali refused to live her life as anything other than absolutely normal. She may have NMO— but NMO did not have her.

Ali has always been so incredibly courageous. But of course she was afraid. She understood the big picture, yet she didn't want to know the details. Or, as she would later say, she wasn't ready to get to know her diagnosis on a first-name basis. She wanted to be able to control the moment and make the choice to ask when she was ready.

And much as I tried to honor her wish, Ali didn't get to make the choice of when to know NMO by name—or the global impact this disease would have on the world through her. That moment happened in the kitchen one day as I sat poring over medical literature. Ali arrived home from school, bouncing in with books under her arm and her tennis bag slung over her shoulder. A piece of mail on the counter happened to state the three letters she had avoided acknowledging all this time.

"Oh," she said quietly, "is this what I have?"

I nodded and reassured her I would do my best to answer any questions she had.

She did not have many. She still needed to take it in and in small sips. Later she would come into her own as an expert, reminding others through her example that knowledge is power. But back then—for that tender moment in time—all she believed and all she wanted to know was that I was going to cure it.

But Ali also knew something else that I hadn't fully considered. Perhaps it came from her intuitive gifts of being able to see beyond that moment into the future. Or from her ability to look past the surface of a reflection—knowing what secrets can be found in the mirror itself.

"You know, Mom," she began, and pointed to all the early work that had already been done to build the Foundation focused on curing NMO. "This isn't just about me and you. It's so much bigger than both of us."

When she said it, my singular focus on saving Ali suddenly expanded into a global vision that had not been there before.

People with rare diseases like NMO often inspire because they are inspired—to contribute, donate, teach, and to help others like them, even those they don't know.

—Dean M. Wingerchuk, MD, MSc, FRCP(C)
Professor and Chair Department of Neurology, Mayo Clinic, Phoenix/Scottsdale, AZ

THE LITTLE FOUNDATION THAT COULD

Ali inspired our family foundation to become something greater. This would not be achieved by magical or wishful thinking. No, this would take bold and decisive action. It would mean standing up to criticism. It would mean giving every idea the opportunity to be heard. It would mean setting a course, measuring progress, and navigating the pitfalls that can otherwise cause voyages—no matter how majestic in purpose—to run aground. The need for our blueprint became all the more necessary. After all, even the greatest goal is simply a wish unless there is a plan.

Time and again, history teaches us that humans are an incredible problem-solving species. Perseverance in the face of all odds emerges as a theme of great achievement. Everyone thought polio was incurable. That stepping foot on the moon was impossible. How many diseases, mysteries, or impossibilities have been cured, solved, or made possible despite daunting challenges?

Our foundation was born of the vision that we could and would cure NMO—for Ali and for every patient like her. The cure was always bigger than just us.

The lessons I learned in my journey from mascara to medicine might not have been obvious to me at first. But as time has gone on, they have proven to be indispensible—in ways that are both personal and universal:

- *Know thyself.* When the universe challenges you, look into yourself first—know your strengths and admit your weaknesses. Doing so will reveal gifts and resources you didn't know you had, or remind you of those waiting silently within you.

- In choosing to trust yourself and lead the charge against the status quo, be prepared to let go of preconceived notions and illusions. Einstein said, "We can't solve problems with the same kind of thinking we used when we created them."

- Wishing and hoping can help inspire action, but they alone will not move one step toward solutions—you must act . . . and with purpose. Plan and act to best put your depths and capacities to work. Movement is critical to survival.

- Be bold. Be brave. Be loud. Strength and resolve get attention. Trust your voice to say "cure" or whatever your mission goal really is. Summon your inner Michelangelo—who urged us all to remember: "The greater risk is not that we aim too high and fail, but that we aim too low and succeed."

- We all have the right to ask *why*—along with *what* or *how* or *where* or *when*. In our DNA resides the power of our intuition and the ability to ask the questions that guide us to hidden answers.

- Understanding that your cause is bigger than just you and yours is a gateway to meaning. You may not know all the dimensions of that meaning when you begin—but if you keep your mind and heart open—you will find the vision to bring your own blueprint for change to life.

My first challenge had been to learn the language of curing a disease. My next step was to find the most brilliant problem solvers from around the world and get them into the same room. We would need a paradigm shift. We would need to change the rules. We would need to build a round table big enough to change the world of NMO.

And it was Ali who gave the Power of Rare to this little foundation that could.

Collaboration has no hierarchy.
The Sun collaborates with soil
to bring flowers on the earth.
—Amit Ray
Enlightenment Step by Step

CHAPTER 3

EVERYONE IN THE ROOM

How do you create what doesn't yet exist? How do you give form to a vision so that others can see it and join together with you to make it a reality? How do you take on the complacency of the status quo and change it for the better?

Those were the kinds of essential questions I had begun asking myself years earlier in my journey as an entrepreneur. And along that path, such questions had opened my eyes to a handful of lasting truths.

One recurring truth is that if you really want to create the change necessary to bring a radical vision to life, it's not enough to think outside the box—or even to destroy the box. The more energy you give the box, the more its walls and boundaries prevent change—and limit your vision. Instead, the challenge is to think as if there were no box at all.

But it is also true that new ideas and those who create them can still respect their predecessors, and even build on them. And often there is an energizing power in the creative tension that results from differing points of view. That's what happens when you get rid of the box and replace it with a blueprint for change informed by multiple perspectives, each important for bringing an ambitious or so-called "impossible" vision to life.

We brought this same philosophy to the field of NMO in a way that would produce more new insights and opportunities to diagnose, treat, and cure this disease in just one decade than had been reached in an entire century prior. We definitely did not do it by the book. Or by the box. We did it by putting patients first and then challenging problem solvers to apply their rare powers of *possible*.

My intuition told me from the start that getting everyone in the room was the first step in our quest to solve NMO. Next, we had to convince all of them that they should be energized to use their areas of expertise— their pieces of the puzzle—to cure this mystery disease. Then we would politely refuse to let them out of the room until they arrived at a solution *together*—to build our strategic priorities with actionable plans.

If we could do that, I knew the process would be revolutionary and the results life-saving.

PLANTING SEEDS IN A DESERT

And so we began.

In the fall of 2008, we held our first-ever Roundtable gathering—an intense daylong event that the Foundation hosted in a small hotel conference room in Beverly Hills. I remember being able to finally catch my breath for the first time since Ali's NMO diagnosis. As dark and uncertain as that period was, I felt at last there was a crack of light breaking through.

We were beginning to find our way out of a bygone era in which NMO had no voice. We were planting seeds in a desert to give life to a long-overdue mission—even if that meant having to reinvent the medical research process while we were at it.

And that takes conviction. You can't control the threats, and you have to weather the storms. Conviction says life will find a way.

Our first Roundtable was a declaration to everyone that we had the conviction to solve NMO. We had among us some of the most renowned names in medicine and science—each with rare expertise—along with a few rising stars who would add their own big, bold ideas to the mix. The business world had taught me the value of including younger thinkers whose energy and outsider status gave them a healthy naïveté to challenge dogma—and whose questions of "*Why not?*" could overpower doubts of "*Why try?*"

When I stood to welcome everyone on behalf of our family and the Foundation, I felt the weight of the moment. All my fears and hopes were concentrated into one pure intention: to solve this disease and save my beautiful daughter—and patients like her. In a room filled with scientific and medical giants, I spoke simply, from my heart to theirs, thanking them and sharing my conviction that together we had begun a collaboration that would forever change the uncertainty of NMO and offer real hope—where there had been so little for so long.

Looking back at the moment, I realize now that we had already defied a few odds. The skeptics had scoffed at the idea that we would succeed in getting the top names from diverse disciplines to sit down and share their prized expertise with one another to solve a rare and orphan disease.

At first, this made no sense to me. From an emotional standpoint, such criticisms seemed absurd. Of course, people should share in the best interests of finding cures. Intellectually, though, I got it, and the realities were more complex. We would need to find innovative ways to overcome traditional barriers to cooperation.

Still, our expectations didn't seem unreasonable. Our mission, rooted in life-and-death urgency, was to devise a science-focused, patient-centered, practical plan to understand the causes of NMO—and find ways to stop it. Our goal was to rapidly advance molecular and cellular knowledge of NMO and to link that knowledge of causes to pioneering cures. Such a purpose seemed obvious and straightforward when we first crafted our strategies and priorities for funding research and came up with our expectations for how there could be and would be collaborative thinking.

All of that was clear. *Except*—there was an issue, a recurring theme I started hearing about in the months leading up to the Roundtable. Apparently, much of the time, medical research had been taking place in an everyone-for-themselves system, with experts hunkered down in their own "secret silos."

Another problem to be solved.

RETHINKING EVERYTHING NMO

I'll never forget my disbelief when I first learned there was no common hub for finding or sharing NMO information. The shock of being in the dark had been terrifying enough. Worse was not being able to reach for the light switch. But the biggest blow was realizing there wasn't any light source yet installed for NMO.

My reaction was a mixed bag of *"Oh, my God, really?"* and *"Well, let's add that to the list of what has to be changed."*

Yes, there were the sparse, outdated one-page "fact sheets" on the Internet that described NMO in nineteenth-century thinking as if all the answers were known: an extreme type of multiple sclerosis from which few recovered or survived. Horrifying.

Otherwise, wherever I looked was a desert barren of detail or direction. No central database for physicians or scientists to access. No national registry. No way of connecting networks of patients to resources or experts or information about promising research that would soon be in motion. There were no NMO-specific conferences or conversations with opinion leaders to even ask the basic questions, let alone find the answers.

For example: How many people had NMO? How many had been misdiagnosed with MS? Where was the outreach to the medical community encouraging better access for testing to see if patients with like illnesses had the NMO-IgG antibody but did not know it? Was NMO really as rare as was thought? Who were the movers and shakers in immunology and drug development who could turn new science into new medicines? These and a thousand other questions pounded in my brain. But there were no answers. NMO was not even really on any public health radar screen. Even at top institutions, there was no communication hotline or system to get the word out. No bulletins to alert healthcare providers when a patient experienced sudden and unexplained blindness or a crippling attack of transverse myelitis—both telltale symptoms of NMO.

How could this be? Patients' lives—*my daughter's life*—hung in the balance. Was it indifference to a rare condition, the complexity of autoimmunity meets brain, or the bureaucracy of an overly complicated healthcare system? Or was it the perception that nothing could be done?

Whatever the reason, I knew we had to build our NMO hub and a communication network that would deliver the latest information to a global patient community, the medical field, and the general public. Urgently. Long before even our first Roundtable, I refused to accept that breakthrough insights into understanding and solving NMO might be lost in some dark laboratory drawer. We needed to tear down the walls and get everyone into the room. We needed the best and brightest out of their silos.

Except—we also had to be pragmatic. Some of the greatest ideas and inventions in history have been conceived and perfected by mavericks working alone in their own way and in their own space.

Realistically, I knew motivating collaboration was not about getting everyone to sit in a circle, hold hands, and share their life's work freely. Not going to happen. Instead, we had to create an atmosphere that brought the best out in each rare thinker—while appreciating their uniqueness. We knew there was no one-size-fits-all way to drive breakthrough research. What we insisted was that each breakthrough be made known to everyone *in time* to save lives. After all, breakthroughs don't fail because they become known too early—they fail because they become known too late.

We also honored independence. And we knew that in the increasingly investment-driven world of research and development, there was mounting pressure on everyone to be competitive—for funding, intellectual property rights, patent ownership, and more. It would have been naive to ignore the fuel of capitalism as a driver of important medical breakthroughs. Besides, I wanted the lone brainiacs and rugged individualists to work as they work best. We absolutely needed those research mavericks too.

But we still had to get them into the room with everyone else. The

challenge was to reframe the old hunker-down mentality that had histori-
cally slowed the pace of real progress—as patient lives were lost. *Except*—I
knew it wasn't enough to just say the old way wasn't working or was in-
efficient. We had to offer a new and different approach—one that would
lead to real, new solutions. Call that a personal problem-solving mantra.

This was a key lesson to be learned—central to our foundation's innovations—that can also be applied to any blueprint for change. Challenging
the status quo didn't mean we had to convince the world of the outmoded
view backward. We just had to show a more promising way forward. Our
job was not to attack the rigid and limiting silo thinking; the challenge
was to illustrate the advantage of real-world and win-win collaboration.
So we would have to offer an alternative, making the sharing of ideas and
information more valuable and more powerful than hiding or hoarding
them. We would encourage and incentivize collaboration—without kill-
ing the independent, competitive spirit essential to breakthroughs.

And so our *room* had to be inviting and inclusive to all. With the right
blend of respect and opportunity, I firmly believed we could get experts
who would never have communicated or collaborated together—and motivate them to solve the problem of NMO.

The question was *how?*

To answer that, I began to envision what can best be called a recipe for
teamwork that would be blended into our overall blueprint. Naturally, the
various "ingredients" needed to be of the highest quality, and they needed
to be adaptable. But more than that—it was *how* they would be combined
that would make all the difference in rethinking everything NMO.

These essential components would evolve and expand but were there
in essence from the start:

1. REDEFINE THE PROBLEM. Even though NMO resides at the in-
   tersection of two great mysteries of the human body—the central
   nervous system and the immune system—these complex systems
   ultimately adhere to more simple truths: pattern recognition,

response, adaptation, memory. By identifying the simplicities within these systems that seemed so complex, new insights would emerge—and from them new stepping stones to solutions.

2. OUTSIDE IN AND INSIDE OUT. As Dr. Yeaman put it: "Experts in a given field may have great knowledge, but that knowledge is often conditioned by their status as insiders." That was why I chose from the start to bring in experts from beyond who were outsiders to the NMO field—to disrupt complacency and dogma, to refresh and invigorate the possible.

3. CULTURE OF OPEN MINDS. Getting diverse experts to the table is a first step. Appreciating their views is another. And stimulating them to think beyond their normal boundaries is yet another. Not much gets done in research when minds are only in agreement. So we had to make it evident to all that new and opposing ways of thinking would not just be tolerated but welcomed and encouraged.

4. FIRST THINGS FIRST. Rather than being paralyzed by the daunting task of trying to decode *every* dimension of the complexity that is NMO, we had to focus on *small, achievable steps* on our greater road to curing the incurable. This key element helped us to concentrate on the handful of critical problems that—if solved—would be the most direct route between making discoveries and saving lives. Solving one problem opens doors to solving other problems.

5. REAL-WORLD REVOLUTION. Collaboration would need carrots as well as diplomatic sticks. It would need mutual recognition and reward—incentives that continually reinforce the power and value in sharing ideas and information. Change needed for curing a real disease would not rest on utopian ideals but in proving that the alternative was achievable, realistic, and offered a better way.

6. A SENSE OF URGENCY. In the lives of NMO patients, every day counts. Each day can be one day closer to a blinding relapse or paralyzing setback—or it can be a breakthrough stride toward

a new treatment and an ultimate cure. We needed to be swift but not rushed, dynamic but never reckless. Everyone needed to know that lives were at stake.

None of these concepts, alone, were radical or new. As an entrepreneur, I had already witnessed how the most successful innovations come from collaboration between members of teams composed of diverse and even unlikely perspectives. The innovative test comes down to how strategies are developed for putting concepts into action—and how those actions synergize in time and place.

You need to be bold and probably a bit audacious to go out looking not just for the best and brightest thinkers in a range of medical specialties but to also expect them to be willing to rethink some of what they already thought they knew.

But that is exactly what we did, and eventually we filled the room.

BRAINS + TRUST = BRAINTRUST

Whenever I think back to the months that led up to that first Roundtable, some of that time remains a blur. We were still in shock, still navigating the daily roller coaster of everything that comes with a life-threatening diagnosis, and still trying to compartmentalize to protect Ali from the fears and uncertainties of a condition she hadn't yet gotten to know by name.

Somehow, I channeled all that turbulent emotion into plowing ahead with the "first things first" part of our mission to get those brightest lights to the table with us.

Early in the summer of 2008, my team and I started compiling a list of some of the most distinguished and brilliant scientists and clinicians who could fit the collaborative bill for our advisory and research teams. Their expertise came from a wide range of backgrounds—including some unexpected places—from specialists versed in NMO and other conditions to outsiders who rarely encountered "rare." We cast a wide net. Sure, we looked for prominent names from the obvious fields—neurology, rheumatology, immunology. But we also went in search of experts from disciplines that may have seemed to be less intuitive for NMO—infection, endocrinology, ophthalmology, epidemiology, and more. We sought out expertise in sectors from brain science to molecular biology to stem cells to pharmacology.

This recruitment process was by no means easy at first.

Members of my newly formed foundation team began by fanning out across the country to attend medical conferences, where they would approach esteemed names in science and medicine about their interest in NMO research. If those approached weren't interested, the next question would be, "Can you suggest an expert who might be?"

I turned over every stone, leveraging every relationship I had to anyone who knew anyone at the highest echelons of medical research. If it meant cold-calling whoever the miracle worker was who might add to our braintrust, I would make that call. Lives were at stake, and the clock was ticking.

In the halls of medical science, this was definitely an uncommon practice. Even so, I had learned from building a business empire from the ground up that sometimes you have to push the envelope—or the microscope—to achieve your most ambitious goals.

That was how we began to assemble the attendees for our first Roundtable. Once we overcame the initial hurdles—especially the reluctance to believe that anything could be done about this mystery disease—a domino effect followed. All it took was one renowned department head to say yes and before long there was another, and over the next few months, we gathered an amazing group of yeses. Between our advisory panel and our lead investigator corps, we soon put together a team that blended the wisdom of experience with the courage of upstart—from Nobel Prize winners to rising stars and from clinical pioneers to scientific trailblazers. No surprise that I called this core of advisors and researchers the Knights of the Roundtable.

We found them or they found us. Rare attracted rare.

I saw that so vividly on the morning of our first round table. No one was there by accident. The faces of each of our small band of revolution-aries—just eighteen at that time—were solemn yet energized as we took our seats at our one large, round table. The symbolism was intentional. With no real or perceived head of the table, every voice and every idea would be equally valued as a contributor to the conversation and the con-clusion. Our model was not about superiority or ego or hierarchy. It was about finding answers together that could not be found individually. Even the veterans who had already been studying NMO were fired up, eager to learn, and unafraid to chime in.

From that morning forward, an NMO alchemy came to life. A med-ical revolution was under way.

THE ENERGY OF "AS IF" THINKING

Back when I was still struggling to put my cosmetics line on the map, I weathered the leanest days by thinking it was "as if" my vision of "making it" was already unfolding—long before it did. I would imagine in vivid detail that I was already reading the story of my success, and one day I would look back at the hard times and appreciate the lessons learned. I even used to envision myself on television, reflecting back on the ups and downs, recounting the struggles to my imaginary mentor—Oprah, of course!

It worked. Wildly. My "no makeup makeup" revolution in natural beauty took off within a week of airing my first infomercial, selling a million dollars of product within days and empowering a generation of women to adopt my mantra: *"When you look better, you feel better—and when you feel better, you can change the world."*

Just as the power of visualizing possibilities worked in the world of cosmetics, I believed it could be applied to curing a disease. But vision is more than just a make-believe hope. It's a distillation of all you value in a goal, and a reference point for all your progress in reaching it. Vision was a cornerstone of our blueprint—essential to the collaborative process by keeping everyone focused on the same goal.

To create the *reality* of that vision, however, the fact-finder in me still had to ask: *how do cures really happen?*

Believe me, that's a question I continue to consume for breakfast, lunch, and dinner—and every moment in between. One of the best answers I've been given is that the medical breakthroughs that have led to miracle cures are not heralded so much with "Eureka!"s (or Oprah's "aha!" moments) but more often with questions than answers, like, "Geez, I never expected to see *that*!?" These moments mark rare instances of serendipity.

A classic example of one of the most important instances of serendipity in medical history happened when Alexander Fleming, a Scottish researcher, conducted an experiment on bacteria but instead saw fungus growing on his petri dish—leading to the discovery of penicillin. Fleming said it this way: "One sometimes finds what one is not looking for. When I woke up just after dawn on September 28, 1928, I certainly didn't plan to revolutionize all medicine by discovering the world's first antibiotic, or bacteria killer. But I guess that was exactly what I did."

The takeaway?

As Dr. Yeaman has put it: "Observing and appreciating the Power of Rare opens up an ocean of cures."

An even more important moral of this story is that you improve the odds of achieving breakthroughs for cures by intentionally and actively creating more opportunities for serendipity—in part by thinking about the challenges in ways that you haven't before.

If we did that, we could then begin to ask an even more visionary question together: *what would a cure for NMO actually look like?*

This would be our way of choosing to think "*as if*" instead of "*as is.*"

Insights about how breakthroughs are achieved can be applied to any challenge: sometimes answers hidden below the surface will only bubble up when you change the conditions that have kept them hidden. By getting everyone in the room and fostering collaboration, that's what we were doing—changing the environment and changing the culture.

But still, there was more coaxing to do to get some of those secrets out of the silos.

HEARTS AND MINDS IN PARALLAX

Getting otherwise disconnected experts around the same symbolic table to rethink solutions was absolutely the necessary and positive first step toward creating our own collaborative culture. But what really bonded us to the same cause and the same vision had to do with connections more powerful than molecules or data: our shared humanity.

I saw that so clearly at our first Roundtable gathering. Nothing about the search for these problem-solving all-stars had been random. Brilliance was important. No question. But there was another kind of scale used to identify the true champions who would alter the course of NMO—one that weighed intuition and inspiration as much as intellect.

Great brains alone were not enough. We needed great hearts as well. We sought those who had a personal connection to NMO, even if they didn't realize it at the outset. We looked for that potent blend of passion and compassion—the drive to care and to cure.

A shared humanity may sound fairly commonplace. Yet, for me, making meaningful connections of the heart has always been one of the most powerful ingredients for successful collaborations. It has been as basic as acknowledging who each expert is as a person, family member, or citizen—separate from their professional job titles—and then appreciating that each has a special calling to be in the room.

With heart, you make it personal for everyone on the mission. For me, true dream teams may boast the greatest minds—the most exceptional talents—but ultimately they are defined by heart.

So I chose from the start to make our story central to our cause and to be honest about my fears, sense of urgency, and love for my daughter. I felt if I could tell our truth and speak from my heart to other hearts, I could engage their minds.

If I could also listen and learn from each person assembled around our Roundtable by sitting in each of their seats and seeing through their eyes, I knew we could make possible an unprecedented collaborative exchange of ideas and insights.

Why does this shared humanity matter?

Because I believe inspiration precedes motivation. No matter how dark and uncertain the situation, to motivate change we must first inspire others to share our conviction that there is a better way—even if it doesn't exist yet. That's why I intuitively sought ways to connect some form of hope or light, interest, or even humor to our shared concerns. Like that moment during the first Roundtable when I admitted out loud, "As soon as we cure this disease, I get to faint."

Laughter followed—as did a show of heads nodding in serious recognition.

I was not the only one in the room dealing with the very human anguish of needing answers to help someone afflicted by a life-threatening, unpredictable illness. Many of the medical researchers who traveled to be part of this day—and who would become almost family—were caring for patients whose conditions ran the gamut from worrisome to critical. These women and men had not chosen their career paths lightly; most genuinely and sincerely did so to serve others and to do their parts to solve medical problems and advance live-changing cures.

And so it remains true from that first Roundtable until today: everyone who has come on board to cure NMO has been personally affected by rare in some way. All have experienced medical mysteries themselves, or had close connections to rare—a patient with a disease seen only once in a career; a family member, a friend, a colleague—*someone*. And for many, it was a life-changing event that set their directional sails on their search for answers both as a profession and a calling.

Despite all the differences in perspective, what we shared was a fiery refusal to accept the conventional stance that a complex medical mystery is unsolvable. In my experience, the first barrier to solving any hard problem is thinking it has no solution. The lesson here is that the first step to finding an answer is *believing an answer exists*.

Our collaboration needed to be more than just exchanging scientific information. It was about taking a leap of faith together that no one could have taken alone. It's a leap of faith that says the unknown can be known and the incurable can be cured—by combining skills and strengths and views and questions to create a new vision.

Dr. Yeaman, one of our core advisors from the beginning, calls this concept *collaborative parallax.*

"What do you mean by 'parallax'?" I asked when he told me about the concept.

He explained that maybe his understanding had something to do with being born in Roswell, New Mexico. Or maybe it was because he studied astrophysics before he went into immunology. Either way, the term "parallax" is often used in the field of astronomy to describe how telescopes located in different places around the world, pointed on the same object, can provide insights that cannot be seen by any single telescope alone.

Ditto for NMO and our research mission: experts from very different places viewing the mysteries of NMO through different lenses that together provide a new view of solutions.

Parallax connects personal to universal to purposeful and lets us each take our own leaps of faith—for whatever our own reasons may be. It is 1 + 1 = 3. Individuals more together than alone.

Hearts, minds, shared humanity—all working in parallax. In this mix, we were all the more fortunate to have true pioneers animate our work. Leaders among leaders.

How do you spot the rare traits that set these innovators apart? In my experience, pioneers are born not taught. They think differently. They're the ones who got rid of the box years ago, or never had it to begin with. They have that sleuthing X factor—and exhibit extraordinary qualities: 1) belief in a purpose greater than themselves; 2) an exceptional ability to view what everyone else views but *see* what no one else sees—through analytical or creative genius (and in the rarest of rare cases, both); 3) empathy for suffering; 4) fearlessness in the face of those who will criticize new and better ways; and 5) a burning internal flame of perseverance.

For someone like me who has not slept much since Ali was diagnosed, I am especially drawn to this last trait. It's a relentless drive that lifts heads off pillows at 3:00 a.m. on a Sunday morning with a breakthrough idea or strategy when everyone else is deep in sleep. It is the fire within those who are always working, brainstorming, questioning—refusing to quit.

I mention the choice to make sleep optional because so many of the researchers who have joined our mission have that drive, many who might just as easily be considered as eccentric as they are enlightened. At one of our meetings, I spoke about this concept with Dr. Alan Verkman, a professor of medicine and physiology from the University of California, San Francisco. He has a special focus in understanding the water channel protein aquaporin-4, believed to be a central target of autoimmunity in NMO.

With his longish hair, I confess to assuming that he was so busy achieving breakthroughs that he just didn't have the time to get it cut. That inspired me to ask him—half joking—"If you stayed up all night, don't you think you could solve this disease and in the morning come up with a new therapy for NMO?"

He paused, then smiled, and with all seriousness simply said, "Yes."

ALL ABOUT PERSPECTIVE

Henry Ford gets the credit for offering an excellent mantra to anyone facing a journey that will be painstaking, winding, and uphill: "Whether you think you can or think you can't—you're right." From the moment I heard the three letters—N-M-O—I began campaigning for a "Yes, we can" reality.

At our first Roundtable, I heard several experts echo that conviction—many agreeing that the prospect of solving NMO together could not have been better timed. It would be "a most promising scientific adventure," according to groundbreaking immunologist Dr. Lawrence Steinman from Stanford University.

Within the year, NMO would no longer be called the "crazy cousin" of autoimmune diseases, as I once heard it described. Doubt would be re-placed with possibility. There were murmurs that NMO was not just con-sidered solvable but was on a much faster track to being cured than, say, MS and other better-known and longer-studied illnesses. Yes, it would take time and money and blood, sweat, and tears—literally. But there is a life-saving difference between thinking *It cannot be cured* and *It can be cured*. It's all about perspective.

Dr. Steinman may have been the first to remind everyone that thanks to the breakthroughs achieved by Dr. Vanda Lennon and the Mayo Clinic team—also present at the first Roundtable—NMO was one of the rare autoimmune diseases to have a distinct biomarker: the autoantibody known as NMO-IgG. That gave us a jump ahead in one of our toughest challenges—figuring out potential triggers for why this identity crisis was taking place at all.

We knew that for certain reasons (yet to be discovered) the misdi-rected immune response targets the aquaporin-4 (AQP4) protein on the surface of astrocytes (star-shaped cells that support the health and func-tion of neurons) in the central nervous system. As we would soon learn, the anti-AQP4 autoantibody (NMO-IgG) is only made when a specific set of immune dominoes is set in motion. And because of the specifics of immune response, our team could study the autoantibody and make major leaps in understanding what are known as the upstream causes (the initiating events or origins of the disease) and downstream effects (the cascade of steps in the process of disease) that lead to the devastating inflammation and demyelination in NMO. Those causes and effects—through all their molecular transactions—would be the basis for our abil-ity to target new drugs and immunotherapies to save and improve patient lives.

Getting everybody into the room to share perspectives was also a chance to get the lay of the land of NMO—known and unknown.

Even though the ultimate cause of NMO was unknown, we were able to ask which research pathways would get us closer to discovering how the disease occurred in different patients in the first place. As pointed out by members of the Mayo team—Doctors Brian Weinshenker, Claudia Lucchinetti, and Sean Pittock—NMO, like many autoimmune conditions, is most likely caused by a combination of factors, and probably different factors in different patients.

Dr. Yeaman offered a perspective that suddenly shifted our thinking. NMO, he began, was similar to a combination lock in which multiple tumblers needed to line up to cause the disease.

Everyone nodded.

Then he added, "But here is the twist: you don't have to solve all the tumblers to prevent the lock from clicking—you just need to solve *one*."

The room went silent. A world of possibilities changed in that moment.

Suddenly, I felt a weight lifting off me. This was the real purpose of getting everyone in the room.

Around the table, we began listing several of the combination lock tumblers. There was the question of genetics. (I had been asking myself whether it could have been *my* genes . . . or was that just my Mom paranoia?). Other tumblers included coexisting autoimmune disease (often the case for many NMO patients), infection, vaccinations (I had specific questions about that), metabolic disorders, endocrine imbalances (or perhaps hormonal changes?), allergies, lifestyle choices, and environmental factors. And what about diet or stress—and beyond?

As little exploration had been conducted into NMO on these many fronts, several of these tumblers presented huge opportunities for research to benefit patients in immediate ways. There was also a growing body of new information offered for public consumption that we could look at. For example, authors T. Colin Campbell, PhD, and Thomas M. Campbell II, MD, had recently published a book called *The China Study: The Most Comprehensive Study of Nutrition Ever Conducted and the Startling Implications for Diet, Weight Loss and Long-Term Health*. In it they looked at how certain foods—and the declining condition of our food supply—could be connected to declining overall health. They also cited studies suggesting that gluten-free diets had significantly benefitted certain autoimmune disease patients. In my view, we had to be open-minded to any potential cause or possible remedy to save my daughter.

Another intriguing report emerging from the medical literature had shown that vitamin D is required for proper immune response. So why not commission research to look at how perhaps abnormalities in vitamin D pathways or other nutrients might be contributing to inflammation in NMO or other autoimmunity?

Not everyone agreed that research into factors such as diet and nutrition was necessarily mission-critical. However, after a back-and-forth, there was consensus that at least looking into these possibilities could be important. The strategy that emerged was that we had to pay close attention to the gut connection and various GI symptoms (nausea, vomiting, excessive hiccups) that sometimes precede or accompany the onset of NMO.

The lesson from this process was important to my blueprint as a reminder that, as Dr. Yeaman phrased it—"Consensus may not mean unanimity." We wanted—we *needed*—the outliers in our midst with strong opinions to state their case—pro and con. We also had to find a balance between near-term urgency to find life-saving treatments and longer-term research that might uncover cures.

Questions we also addressed were about factors of geography, race, and gender. Why, for instance, did NMO afflict so many more females than males—with a ratio of up to seven females to one male? It didn't take a rocket scientist to realize that gender was a factor in NMO. Without exact answers, we still could infer that maybe it was worth looking into a hormonal component to relapses—a topic that would lead to multiple research avenues.

Hammering out perspectives about these questions—never before asked in a room with this much brainpower devoted to NMO—led me to a simple conclusion: *if the cause of the problem is multifactorial, the solution has to be as well, right?*

Maybe—maybe not.

Either way, we needed to establish baseline questions that could then become even more fine-tuned. Dr. Weinshenker raised several: "Why does NMO selectively target the optic nerves and spinal cord? Why are its attacks so severe and its course so aggressive with frequent yet unpredictable clusters of attacks?"

Dr. Lucchinetti answered by highlighting the need to identify causes upstream rather than downstream, where all the damage was done, because in her opinion, "There's some very critical immune-regulatory events at the get-go. If you can define those and dissect them, then you could maybe get in before you've gone down an irreversible path." As it turned out, a year later her work would move her to add: "I see reversibility in the disease." Her stance was clear-cut: if NMO could be understood and arrested in its earliest stage, it could be reversed—and if it could be reversed, then no patient would have to suffer relapses or life-changing disability.

PREPARING FOR A MARATHON NOT A SPRINT

Whenever I am feeling overwhelmed by the distance still to go in the quest for an ultimate cure for NMO, I have to think back to that first Roundtable and recall just how far we've come. Many of the questions originally posed have been answered. At that meeting, we were still grappling with just how many NMO patients were out there—and where in the world were they? Also: why had so many patients come to these top clinicians with misdiagnoses of MS or other autoimmune diseases that presented with similar symptoms—and what could be done about it? Another big one for me: who was at risk of being struck by NMO—and how could we prevent it before it happened?

I remember the Mayo's Dr. Sean Pittock conservatively estimating that the majority of NMO patients up to that time had been initially misdiagnosed, often going for months and even years on end before getting the right diagnosis. Surveys of NMO patients would later suggest that it might be as high as 90 percent.

Less than a year later, a breakthrough study would give us a clearer picture of the numbers and the impact of accurate diagnosis on benefit-ting patients' lives, with NMO and MS alike. In a press release from the Mayo Clinic, also reprinted in a handful of medical journals and publica-tions, the new understanding was:

Thousands of Neuromyelitis Optica (NMO) patients are po-tentially being misdiagnosed with Multiple Sclerosis (MS), ac-cording to Mayo Clinic Neurologist Sean Pittock, MD, largely due to lack of awareness of NMO within the medical commu-nity. Dr. Pittock shared this finding with more than 50 of the world's leading doctors and medical researchers—from Harvard to Oxford—who gathered at the 2009 NMO Roundtable Con-ference, sponsored by the Guthy-Jackson Charitable Foundation.

Dr. Pittock came to his conclusion based on ongoing research at the Mayo Clinic. Of the 1,200 blood samples that are sent to the Mayo Clinic's neuroimmunology laboratory for NMO an-tibody (NMO-IgG) testing each month, approximately 70 new patients test positive for NMO, which is surprisingly high con-sidering it is believed to be a rare disease. Of the 70 patients who have the NMO antibody, Dr. Pittock has found that a majority were previously thought to have MS. . . .

Dr. Pittock believes that part of the reason for the lack of awareness of NMO is that there was no biomarker until recently, and traditionally, NMO was considered by many in the medical and research communities to be a form of MS, a difficult disease to diagnose. Recent clinical and pathological studies now support the concept that NMO is a distinct disease from MS. . . .

At the conference, Mayo Clinic Neurologist Dean Winger-chuk, MD, also reported that the prevalence and incidence of NMO have not been firmly established. . . .

That is why the Guthy-Jackson Charitable Foundation is launching a significant medical education campaign to ensure that doctors nationwide are aware of the differences between MS and NMO. Doing so will help patients get the appropriate treatments and will help more researchers collect the best data in their pursuit of a cure.

Within a few more years, as our braintrust and patient community expanded globally, we would be able to establish that NMO is *50 percent more common* than originally believed. More and more, we would be taking on the status quo to prove why rare matters to everyone. Slowly but surely, we would be learning NMO might not be so ultra-rare after all.

In the meantime, we had also recognized at our first Roundtable that a collaborative effort would need to focus on modernizing and defining the diagnostic criteria for NMO. The blood test was an essential tool for diagnosis but was not failsafe, as not every patient who had NMO tested positive for the NMO-IgG autoantibody. For this reason, one of the advances in the field would be the recognition of NMOSD, or NMO Spectrum Disorder, which included distinct patients who seemed to have NMO without NMO-IgG.

Dr. Brian Weinshenker underscored why establishing definitive criteria was so important when he insisted, "The key is making the diagnosis accurately—and *early*. That's the single most important thing as far as treatment."

Even though I knew this was going to be a marathon and not a sprint, I admit that even at that first meeting there were revelations about the sheer complexity and cruelty of NMO that threatened to send me down a rabbit hole of fear. Probably the toughest moment out of the first Roundtable discussion was hearing the viewpoint expressed by more than a few of our experts that—in spite of their conviction that NMO was solvable—the destination of an absolute cure would not be reached overnight.

Decoded: we had a long and arduous marathon climb ahead. Instead what was recommended was to focus on interim goals—to achieve a "functional" cure, starting with safer and more effective treatments.

Deep breath.

This was the reality, and I never expected an immediate fix. Bracing myself to ask what could be hoped for sooner rather than later, I then heard welcome news. Many around the table agreed in theory about a possibility for prevention that made total sense. If you could find a way to prevent attacks from happening, in effect it would arrest the disease and prevent the terrible toll that NMO takes. That was what was meant by a functional cure.

Mission-critical. No doubt about it—research into how attacks were being triggered and how to head them off at the pass had to be high on our priority list.

Another strong impression that I took away from our first and subsequent meetings was that collaboration—in medicine as in business—had to be orchestrated in keeping with the different personalities and styles of all collaborators. That's because the motivation to share and collaborate aloud often varies greatly from person to person, and from sharer to sharer.

Some share to build consensus, others to challenge it. Some share to educate altruistically, others to elevate their expertise or brand their problem-solving identity. Others share as if putting words to new thoughts—to hear their ideas take form or float possibilities. Others argue to provoke deeper thinking. Others edit the ideas they hear from the room at large and then raise them up a notch.

So how do the best ideas rise above the rest to become life-saving innovations? That's where leadership comes in, I believe—along with the need to empower certain leaders in the room to take ownership of particular projects.

Frankly, it would have been naive to assume that a medical breakthrough would arrive simply by me holding up a conductor's baton and allowing all the voices to come together in a Hallelujah chorus. Nice thought—not realistic. Besides, disagreement and discord can be desirable when in search of truths.

One of our solutions was to encourage collaborators to form small teams, each focused on a big idea. We knew that in each of those groups, leaders would emerge. From principal investigators to advisory captains, every great effort requires enlightened minds who are capable and willing to take the helm and harness the brilliance of other contributors. These are the rarest leaders of leaders who have a knack for making sure all the members of the team have their own winning, unique roles to play in the collaborative effort.

Exchanges in the room don't always produce an immediate reaction or debate leading to a conclusion, yay or nay. Sometimes it's about listening, digesting, and then having the discovery later on. On this subject, I have a vivid recollection of our first Roundtable and watching a proverbial lightbulb go off for one of the youngest members of our team—Dr. Michael Levy, then just finishing his residency at Johns Hopkins—as he began to make scientific notes and diagrams on a notepad. He leaned in to the table, as did everyone else. Whatever his early concept was, I didn't know. I can tell you that in addition to choosing to focus on NMO in his thriving career, Dr. Levy would go on to develop a patent for a vaccine-type treatment aimed at preventing NMO attacks. These advances were catalyzed by his receiving funding for his research from our foundation. And through the hands-on help of our advisors—Dr. Terry Smith (Professor of Ophthalmology and Visual Sciences at University of Michigan's Kellogg Eye Center) and Dr. Yeaman—Dr. Levy was able to parlay his research into a large grant from the NIH.

Most foundations don't choose to invest time or resources in helping grantees go beyond the scope of their funding. We have a different perspective. We want all our investigators and clinicians to succeed wildly—and to reap the rewards of credit and distinction that follow. We just want NMO to be cured, regardless of who gets the credit. That's always been an essential part of our blueprint. It has proven that the collaborative spirit can exist side by side with the individual passion for conquering the unknown. The moral of the story is that by fostering both, we could move much faster than the traditional research time clock usually allowed—*and* we could empower everyone in the room to play a role and go the distance together.

And then we all win—patients, above all. This was all by design.

INCENTIVIZING RARE SOLUTIONS

When Bill and I first confronted the reasons investigators and institutions were averse to collaboration or cautious about sharing too much of their proprietary research, we recognized that much of the system for funding research needed a medical makeover.

Did somebody say makeover? That was definitely in my wheelhouse. And as an entrepreneur and marketing pioneer, Bill also brought a world of insights into our planning about how to incentivize innovation—i.e., change the culture.

As outsiders, however, we had to walk a respectful line. We understood that collaboration was known to be fraught with ego and issues of legality and intellectual property, not to mention the bureaucratic complexities of institutions and agencies alike.

Certain skeptics who considered themselves "in the know" had also cautioned us against various pitfalls. It seemed there were unspoken disconnects between those who fund research with certain expectations and the pure scientists who are only in search of truth in discovery. Not a situation that would delight the funders or founders. We wanted brave new research, but we also wanted it turned into beneficial new medicine. So, on the one hand, we were drawing from our entrepreneurial perspectives, but on the other, we were also philanthropists who cared above all about real results that would ultimately improve and save lives. Test tubes were the means—lives were the ends.

The creative challenge was to incentivize collaboration without getting rid of healthy competition. We had to put our money where our mouths were to catalyze bold new science, first and foremost. Ours became a hybrid model that blended academic rigor with business reward—a competitive process that tied collaborative results to getting paid. We asked investigators to present novel, thoughtful studies, the progress in which would be readily shared in our Roundtables and other conferences.

We looked for a compelling proof of concept that would: a) be

mission-critical to advance the causes of NMO at the molecular and cellular levels; and b) could turn that understanding into new and better
therapies and ultimate cures for NMO patients.

And the work couldn't duplicate other research that was under way.
In many cases, we encouraged groups from completely different parts of
the world to work in partnership. Skype and email and the rest of the
digital network would be the meeting space. Of course, there could still
be competition, but it would be healthy and transparent, not cryptic or
cutthroat. This added excitement, even intrigue: Who was doing what?
Who would make the next breakthrough and up the ante for all? Far from
being a deterrent, our collaborative/competitive model was what many
called "every researcher's dream."

As philanthropists, Bill and I made the choice from the start to devote
significant but heartfelt resources to desperately needed research. From
our inception as funders, our policy has been to allow researchers and
their institutions to retain the patents and intellectual property ownership
connected to discoveries enabled by our funding. For us, this is a win-
win model—an incentive that goes to the benefit of the investigators and
institutions *and* our mission, because of the advances achieved. We have
not only encouraged our funded researchers to keep proprietary interests
in terms of publishing their findings, but we actually made it one of our
requirements. And making their results public was a requirement as well.
Even if the study didn't work, per se, or resulted in negative findings, those
data still had to be reported—to educate the field and advance the cause.

These incentives have put NMO on the medical map in ways we
couldn't have anticipated. Over the last five years, as just one example of
the significance of how our research has gone viral, the number of NMO
publications tripled. Today, there are more than 3,700 papers on NMO,
and counting. The number of times these papers have been cited in scientific and medical journals has exploded from less than 200 in 2007 to
more than 9,000 in 2016.

In our guidelines, we wanted our grantees to think ahead in terms of accountability and the ongoing impact of their work product—which is another way to stay out of an exclusive silo mentality down the road. We asked for: a) a clear pathway for NMO patient benefit; b) specific milestones to be accomplished in each period of the project; c) a data sharing plan; and d) a specific plan to obtain follow-on research funding beyond the GJCF (e.g., NIH or equivalent agency or commercial funding). Anyone could apply and everyone would follow the same rules.

In the business world, the term "tranching" means to set dollar values for goals reached—performance "carrots," or incentives for hitting stated benchmarks. From the start, our grant awards were set up as tranched—just as in a business deal. That meant ongoing funding of all grant types would be dependent on documented accomplishment of milestones in the prior review period, typically every quarter or six months.

Another rare feature of our funding process has been maintaining a deep bench of a diverse group of advisors from varied backgrounds—who don't necessarily specialize in NMO but who have been global groundbreakers in other disciplines. To avoid any real or perceived conflicts of interest, advisors could not be research grantees at the time of their tenure on our grant-awarding jury.

And this is where our foundation steps out of any traditional funding box. Our advisors not only make recommendations to us as founders, but if an investigator asks, members of the advisory board offer their expertise to help refine proposals—making sure the project meets expectations for critical path results. That's really unheard of and worth repeating in case it hasn't rung a bell yet with anyone looking to incentivize breakthrough research: our expert grant reviewers *actually get in the trenches to help investigators design the most informative studies that will give them the best chance of funding.*

Our position was that we wanted success. Rather than reject proposals outright that fell short of our needs, we opted to invest resources of time and brainpower to overcome limitations and realize potential. Rather than fostering an environment of defensive criticism, we chose to fuel a platform for developing cures. Collaboration—*squared.*

This theme continues even as studies are under way. Call it friendly course correction. If a study becomes stalled or too diffuse or has strayed from its original focus, we will work with the investigators on the fly if necessary—always with the goal of making sure we're moving faster and closer to discoveries that can make a difference in a patient's life and well-being.

Yep, we employ appealing carrots *and* friendly but firm sticks to remind everyone—*check your egos at the door if you want to find cures.*

ONE FOR ALL AND ALL FOR ONE

As for the competitive selection process, we pay strict attention to how proposed research might best address the most urgent needs of patients. To determine what those needs really are, I consult as many of our stakeholders as I can—especially patients, caregivers, and clinicians—and also draw from my own intuition and experience as Ali's mother. Occasionally, rather than waiting for grant applications, my team and I have reached out to investigators to ask for submissions to address unmet questions already percolating.

If the best didn't come to the NMO mountain, we brought the mountain to them.

I've had a special interest, for example, in research that contributes to ways that medicine can become more personalized. Custom care as opposed to one-size-fits-all. It's great when discoveries can be applied with equal benefit to the masses. However, as I've learned from looking through the lens of NMO, I believe the greatest benefit to all will come from research and clinical care that treats each patient as one of a kind.

Vaccines—which we know save countless lives—are a case in point. In a universe of rare, there should be better ways of knowing who may benefit most from certain vaccines and of knowing who might be at risk for adverse reactions. Clearly, this is a conversation that should be explored and discussed thoughtfully between patients, families, and doctors.

As NMO—along with certain other autoimmune diseases—targets women predominantly, I have chosen to spur studies into risk factors of pregnancy, both for the mother and the child. We would learn, for example, that there is a significant difference in pregnancy risks for women with NMO versus women with MS. Why that is and what more can be done about it require ongoing research. What we do know is that medical practitioners want the tools and resources to provide custom care to all patients—especially those in the higher risk groups.

It would be a huge understatement to say it's never easy for me to hear the results of research we sponsored that may not be what I want or hoped to learn. At a recent mini-conference on NMO that we sponsored, I was asked to speak after hearing what the higher risks can be for pregnant women with NMO. During the presentation, I sat in the last row, next to Bill, holding my breath and never forgetting for an instant that I'm Ali's mom. As I stood to comment, I had to summon that survivor piece of myself to find the light and speak to that fear in front of a room of researchers. What I could offer was my gratitude for them never giving up and my will to inspire them to ask questions and find answers to change the very concerning reality that we'd just learned. To engage the energy of their own "as if" thinking.

Meanwhile, regardless of whether a study has been propelled by us, every proposal submitted to us goes through the same rigorous process.

Once our advisors make their recommendations, Bill and I review them. Not only do we assess merit based on science but also on value. Usually, we have agreed with advisors, and sometimes we've asked for further information of the prospective grantee. One helpful method for decision-making that I've borrowed from Bill is what the marketing world calls "USP"—the Unique Selling Proposition. Bill applies the USP test as a measure of what makes a product or project or idea not only unique but highly capable of catalyzing attention on a larger scale.

Using my own version of a USP, I've learned to evaluate proposals with an eye to how that pioneering science could ultimately yield life-changing medicine and how it could give hope to patients and create a buzz that says, "Yes, we have promising breakthroughs coming down the pike." The USP might also tell me how the study could offer new talking points whenever I reach out to those who have not yet connected to why they should care about rare. It's a bite-sized version of the proof of concept—the innovator elevator pitch. The USP matters as much in medical research as in business because it could help put us on the map, priming the well and building awareness that we are uncovering answers that might impact other diseases too. The USP can even predict how headlines might be made that can reach distant shores where cures might be found.

Sometimes the decision of whether or not to fund a proposal has come down to a much more intangible process. In some instances, it was a matter of wanting to hear if an investigator was genuinely committed to the mission of solving NMO. Even if we had already decided to award the money, I've chosen to first sit down with that potential grantee—face to face—and ask simple questions from the heart. They could be as basic as, "How is this science going to help my daughter and all NMO patients?" and "Can you explain to me how this research will get us to a better treatment and an eventual cure?"

By putting my questions in such deeply personal terms, the responses become all the more personal. Maybe that's not how science is supposed to work. But I have found that when you ask the smartest gals and guys in the room to unlock solutions nobody else has managed to unlock, you're making it personal for them too—and that can be a more powerful incentive than any dollars or degrees.

It's important to add that many of our grant proposals have not been "cold" submissions. When we get them, they may already be familiar to our advisors and foundation team. That's because of the Roundtable or meeting where everyone was in the room together—and where many significant studies have first been conceptualized.

Those moments are profound to witness, when someone around the table asks, "Wow, has anybody ever looked into that?" and someone else says, "No, but that's exactly what we should do . . ." And suddenly they are discussing the experimental design. Such encounters happen frequently when rare thinkers convene—thanks to free-form exchanges or provocative questions asked in the midst of breakout sessions that we include for brainstorming or during social chats while breaking bread.

By bread I mean just that. Yes, we outdo ourselves when it comes to what we serve at every meal and snack.

The more serious point for me, and how this connects to a blueprint for change, has come from lessons learned about cultivating the environment of the room itself. Metaphorically—whether it is what you serve, how you set the table, or how you create inclusion and welcoming in seating—the meal is more than just the food. Every sense can matter.

For example, we began hosting scientific summits in the midst of our avocado farm–meets–horse ranch that's away from the noise of the rest of the world at the top of a mountain near Santa Barbara. My feeling was that if we were seeking to foster collaboration, we could nudge it along by getting the brightest minds away from their clinics and labs and out into nature. That's my aesthetic, too, more than anything—that putting people in beautiful settings can be conducive to more creative, even breakthrough, thinking.

Wherever our various meeting sites have been, each has reflected my idea of a large extended *family room*. By design—and yet another strategy for engaging hearts and minds—these varied settings give permission to everyone at the table to think as boldly, rarely, and collaboratively as possible.

Of course, at the time of our first Roundtable we were a far cry from getting everyone into the room who needed to be there. In fact, we were still missing the presence of the most important part of our NMO family—our patients.

To remedy that, it was Ali who by our next Roundtable would provide the inspiration to make sure that the cure would be brought into the room.

AND THEN THERE WERE TWO

In that same summer of 2008, when I was immersed in educating myself in the intricacies of the immune system so I could become a "Dr. Mom," I was also desperate to locate other NMO patients and learn firsthand of their experiences and challenges. That quest became even more urgent as we began to build the hub for our patient community—a reference point and source of information, hope, and guidance for NMO patients, families, caregivers, and healthcare partners.

So there would be no more NMO "orphans," I wanted this hub to be a true home—a warm, inviting, and meaning-rich place of belonging. Based on our own experience, we knew all too well the loneliness of not knowing where to turn for the most basic of information. We wanted this home to offer the resources and community for rare patients not to feel alone—to know someone out there really cared.

Somehow, in those early days, I expected I'd have to travel a great distance to meet the first NMO patient I would come to know after Ali. To my surprise, I would soon be introduced to a young woman—whom I will call Janis (to honor privacy)—who lived in Los Angeles—and who was hosting a fund-raiser to raise money so she could travel to India to receive an experimental stem cell treatment. Though controversial, the treatment had a chance of helping at a time when she had recently suffered a serious NMO relapse.

I'll never forget watching Janis—beautiful and independent—greeting her guests. She was dressed in a sari for this culturally themed event that was complete with Indian food and sitar music. I was so new to the world of a condition that so little was known about, I couldn't help asking myself if this was where my journey would lead—me astride an elephant climbing up a mountaintop in India to find the secret cure. If that was to be, that's what we would do for Ali and Janis and all the other patients I had yet to meet.

When I introduced myself and told Janis about my daughter and the Foundation we were forming, Janis immediately hugged me and said, "Call on me any time. *Please.*"

I listened to her speaking to the small crowd that had come to support her that night. That's when the question first struck me—what exactly was happening inside both these rare patients? What was it about Janis and Ali that connected them in a cellular or genetic way and that led to the same rare condition? Was there some common thread in their experiences or in the environment that had triggered the same illness in each of them? These were questions, I realized, that would ultimately be answered by experts and patients together.

Six years earlier Janis had been doing volunteer work overseas when she suddenly suffered the loss of vision in one eye. She was treated with steroids, which brought her sight back, and was soon misdiagnosed with MS. Back at home, she suffered another attack of optic neuritis in the other eye, followed next by her first spinal transverse myelitis attack. Finally, a neurologist questioned the diagnosis of MS and suggested Janis could have Devic's disease.

Here was this vibrant, lovely young woman whose misdiagnosis had led to ineffective treatment that had resulted tragically in permanent vision loss. "If I had known what it was, I might have been able to save my sight," she told the guests at her fund-raiser that night. "That's why getting the word out is so important."

Those words, so matter-of-fact, seared themselves into my consciousness. Nobody should ever have to lose their eyesight or their mobility—or worse—because information somehow couldn't make it into the hands of medical providers who truly want to give the best, most appropriate care they can.

"We have to do something about that," I told Janis, and promised the work of the Foundation would address the concerns she raised. And more.

Afterward, Janis would go on to play a prominent and vocal role as a patient advocate on behalf of our foundation—helping spread the word to fellow patients and practitioners alike. She was one of us, overcoming her own struggles to help build our virtual and real community home for everyone impacted by NMO.

First there was one patient—and then there were two.

And just at the same time that rare was attracting rare to form our research braintrust, more patients began to find us, and we began to find more of them. A vision of getting everyone into the same room was starting to materialize. But not fast enough.

NMO patients are rare. But rare does not mean unimportant, uninformative, or uninspiring. This rare disease, and people affected by it, have taught me invaluable lessons about the nervous system, autoimmunity, and the human spirit. As a result, I am continually inspired to work harder to answer the questions that can bring a potential cure one step closer.

—Jeffrey L. Bennett, MD, PhD

Gertrude Gilden Professor for
Neurodegenerative Disease Research,
Departments of Neurology & Ophthalmology
Associate Director of Translational Research,
Center for Neuroscience,
University of Colorado, Denver

NO MORE ORPHANS

Meeting Janis only reinforced what I had learned from Ali—that empowered patients had pivotal roles to play in solving NMO. Now they needed their own seats at the table.

I had to make sure we had the resources and strategies in place to pave the way. Questions were raised that I hadn't considered before. In addition to supplying information to the newly diagnosed, how could we best respond to the needs of patients already diagnosed? How could I constructively rattle the cages of the medical system at large to propel speedier and more accurate diagnoses for the patients who were being misdiagnosed? What were the best ways to get information out to everyone about a rare—or maybe not so rare—disease that wasn't yet on their radar?

In the beginning, Bill asked if expanding outreach to patients would be getting ahead of ourselves—going outside our mission to prioritize research. My response was simply, "Patients *are* our mission."

And he agreed. Without question, finding the vital answers to help save lives of patients was the purpose of the Foundation and all its research. It just made sense that we had to go further by creating a community where patients did not feel isolated from all the other components. The more educated and engaged our entire NMO family, the more collaborative all our efforts would be. Patients, empowered by rare, would be our most valued detectives.

Among the many resources we were in the midst of developing, Ali was the first to suggest that our website include a newsletter she chose to call the *Spectrum.* As NMO is in fact a spectrum disorder—because there are diverse variations of the disease—the name was fitting. I loved that it also honored the rainbow spectrum diversity of patients who had already become part of our NMO community. Their ages and socioeconomic backgrounds ran the gamut—from the youngest pediatric patients to adolescents, young adults, and women and men in midlife and older. NMO, an equal-opportunity offender, didn't discriminate between rich or poor, or between black/white/Latino/Asian or any other cultural groups. The *Spectrum*, led by Ali, who volunteered to serve as its first editor in chief, could not have come at a better moment for connecting patients.

Her next suggestion?

"Mom, wouldn't it make sense for patients to also take part in the Roundtable discussions? You have all the top experts there—we could ask questions of them, and they could ask questions of us." After all, she went on to explain, "Patients are the *real* authorities."

Would that mean inviting patients to attend an afternoon session at what we were planning to hold as a two-day Roundtable event for our second-year gathering?

No, Ali insisted. "We should have our own day." And before I could question or contemplate how to proceed, she went on, "And we'll call it *Patient Day.*"

Boom—that was that. Patient Day it was.

And so, in 2009, we brought fifty-six members of our NMO community—patients, parents, spouses, and caregivers—to the first annual NMO Patient Day. We covered their flights, their hotel rooms, their taxis, and their meals. We wanted their focus to be entirely about belonging, and we wanted them to experience a kind of homecoming.

To this day, I feel privileged to have tearfully witnessed the exchanges between patients as they arrived at our check-in desk and began to introduce themselves to one another. It was as if they had walked into the sunlight, blinking in disbelief, after having lived in the dark alone for so long. Many had never known anyone else with their same diagnosis. Now we were becoming family. No longer isolated. No more orphans.

The day was just as emotional for the researchers who were there to find answers—challenged and thrilled by the questions the patients asked them.

Dr. Benjamin Greenberg of the University of Texas Southwestern—and Ali's personal NMO doctor for many years—was quoted in the *Spectrum* as saying, "It never ceases to amaze me how powerful human interaction can be. Listening to the stories of patients and families living with NMO reminded me and the other clinician scientists why it is we are working to end this condition. It also reminded me that we are partnered with one of the most dedicated and passionate groups of patients in the world."

At the Patient Session, Dr. Greenberg and Dr. Bruce Cree from the University of California, San Francisco, took questions from patients that I had never heard posed. "How do you know you are having a relapse, and how do you tell if it is going to be mild or bad?" one asked. Dr. Cree spoke about how to differentiate between a mild attack and a severe one, and at what point to consult with your neurologist. Another patient asked, "Is there any research going beyond stopping the disease, to repair the damage done by attacks?" Dr. Greenberg described the new work being done in cell therapies—including new uses of stem cells for regenerating the myelin sheath of the optic nerve and the spinal cord "as long as the *wire* [nerve] is still intact."

Later that first Patient Day, I was interviewed by Sandy Banks of the *Los Angeles Times*. This was a breakthrough of sorts when you consider that NMO had been essentially unknown just a year earlier—and the fact that rare diseases face a monumental challenge at gaining major press coverage. When Sandy asked me why we chose to "pick up the tab for scientists to be flown in from around the world and patients from around the country," I emphasized the power of connection.

"Can you imagine—in this day and age when everybody's got a support group—for these people to feel so alone? I wanted them to be able to sit down together, talk to one another," I answered. "That alone was worth everything."

Sandy went on to write about why connecting to rare mattered—having been inspired by meeting Winona Davis. A single mother from Rialto, California, Winona—wrote Sandy—was "raising two daughters with NMO. The oldest, now twenty, got her first symptoms at nine. She spent her tenth birthday hospitalized; doctors couldn't figure out why she couldn't see. Since then, she has battled paralysis and blindness, off and on, traumatized not just by the severity of her symptoms, but by their unpredictability."

This beautiful mother of two daughters with NMO said that until Patient Day, "we felt like we were aliens."

Winona told the *Los Angeles Times* about the sisterhood of NMO mothers that had also been created that day. Here was where I found my belonging, too:

Victoria knows how frightening it is, how helpless the disease can make a mother feel. You don't sleep, you can't think. . . . You can't even tell your child what's wrong. All you can do is try and comfort them.

From comfort to empowerment, solidarity to action, we were becoming a community. That was always the point of getting everyone in the room.

Ali described how it felt to be part of that community when she wrote from her editor desk at the *Spectrum* in early 2010:

Dear Friends,

2009 was a great year. Now I don't mean to brag, but I got straight A's on my report card (junior year in high school . . . not too shabby), I became captain of my tennis team (co-captain, and for next season, but still) and, to top it all off (I know this is going to sound cheesy like the bulk of my last letter, but stay with me on this,) I discovered a new awareness, a different perspective of myself I had never noticed before.

The Symposium in November really opened my eyes to a community I was previously ignorant to associate myself with. The amount of love and support I felt from every individual at that conference was truly awe-inspiring and gave me an even better outlook for this whole thing we've all come to know as NMO. Strangers. People I had never met before had heard of me, wanted to meet me, or were somehow linked to me in this bizarre and funny chain of fate we are creating. We joined together to form one perfect, unified bond that was not once broken throughout our entire time together.

For those of you who couldn't attend, for whatever reason, good or bad, I strongly recommend attending in the future. I am not a fan of science and dread going to Chemistry on a daily basis (no offense, Mr. Kelleher), but the Patient Day wasn't about the science. It was about connecting with people just like me, dealing with what I'm dealing with and even feeling what I'm feeling. No one else can relate to me the way they can.

I guess that was my highlight of 2009, believe it or not, because this "disease" has really been a, not exactly fun, but revealing experience. I've discovered how many people care about me and how profoundly I care for them. We are a small group, but a mighty one. We all create a collective unit, and together, we will become known as the little community that could, can, and will.

Yours Truly,

Ali Guthy

The experience of getting everyone into the room together had taught me one of the most important truths about our work to date and to come: that the cure I was so determined to achieve *for* NMO patients would come from contributions made *by* NMO patients.

Patients were our purpose, *and* they held the secrets—the X factors—to the cure. It was contained within them—in their cells, their blood, their stories, their struggles and sacrifices.

Looking back, I know we hadn't yet built the machine that would catapult us closer to that cure and that would quickly begin to save lives by achieving speedier and more accurate diagnoses. But we had done something few believed possible—we had brought together a diverse assortment of problem solvers. Somewhere in our midst, already, was the cure.

So much was swirling in my head and my heart in those first fifteen months of our foundation's existence. In retrospect, I believe many aspects of our theoretical blueprint began to take form without my conscious interference. It was as if there were a natural force and we had found a way to tap into its momentum. What has become evident since that time is how the values that influenced our vision early on were the best predictors of what was to come. Patients first—purpose-focused. Today, I see how those lessons in values apply not just to solving NMO but to any endeavor seeking to unite many for a greater purpose:

- All world-changing collaborations combine hearts and minds, all connected by the common bond of shared humanity. No matter how different your viewpoints, when you open your hand and lower your shield—putting down your spear and baring your heart—true transformation begins.

- Every modern innovation and every rare solution to our most pressing problems have been first conceived by someone willing to see, think, and act "as-if" rather than "as-is."

- If you want to motivate others to share knowledge and work toward a common cause, appreciate that they are different. Whatever fuels their motivation or provides their incentive—for personal gain or to help save the world—it's all good.

- There is real power in the willingness to break the old rules that no longer serve you or your cause—as long as you have better rules that others can believe in.

- When you combine vision with conviction, a new element is formed that can connect hearts and minds to the same mission. And this precious metal can bring to life that which once only existed in your imagination.

- Outside-the-box thinking is still defined by the box. If you really want to shake up the status quo—release the box—just let it go.

- Impatience—combined with courage and care—can be a virtue. Especially when lives are at stake.

This last valuable lesson was especially on point for me when I could well see that time wasn't on our side. Weirdly, we would have to come up with our own clockworks—our own machinery that would accelerate right alongside the research breakthroughs. We would need to use what we learned as fast as we learned it if we were to save lives.

And thanks to the rare thinkers and doers and believers on our team, that's what we were about to do.

Activism that challenges the status quo,
that attacks deeply rooted problems,
is not for the faint of heart.

—Malcolm Gladwell

CHAPTER 4

BUILDING A CURE MACHINE

Curing a disease is not for wimps.

Even before the ink was dry on our foundation charter, that was something I knew instinctively. And it has served as a mantra ever since—a reminder that has kept me on my feet, especially on those fearful days when all I've wanted to do was curl up in a fetal position in the corner.

Now that we'd gotten everyone into the room and had created incentives for sharing, the greater challenge was figuring out how to translate all that brilliance and life-saving science and patient insight into the moving parts of a real-world, practical delivery mechanism for change. Such was the vision for our cure machine.

Questions and challenges abounded. Not just *what* had to be done— but *how*. How did we connect and synchronize our many different moving parts? How would we overcome the challenges of rare—to map the "where" and "when" and "who" of NMO around the world? How could we get enough blood and data to our researchers when the patient population was so small? How could we help educate the medical community to end the nightmare of misdiagnosis? How could we constructively rattle the cages of the medical establishment to speed more accurate diagnoses for new patients? How could we best respond to the needs of the newly diagnosed? How would we engage industry to invest time and resources in treating and curing this rare disease? And until then, what were the needs of those who had been living with NMO for much of their lives?

These were only some of the challenges before us. What we had to build couldn't be any kind of conventional system or process. Why so ambitious? Because if our machine worked, we knew that the field of NMO would change radically and rapidly. So we had to invent and then put into practice a streamlined system of strategies and actions that could respond to change and overcome obstacles we didn't even know existed yet—as they arose. We had to reshape time. Our cure machine had to be progressive and adaptive.

Or put more simply—necessity had to become the mother not only of invention but also of implementation. When lives are at stake, you rise to the challenge or you fall down. No passes given to the faint-hearted.

Don't get me wrong. There was nothing about what we were up against that was easy or that didn't scare me most of the time. No question. My solution, rather than pretend this was going to be easy, was to take all that fear and uncertainty and distill it into my personal Rx to keep going. The fire inside of me would have to fight the fire outside of me.

On a quest to stop a killer on the loose, I could not be in denial that I was afraid. But I still couldn't be a wimp. Problem-solving, fearful though I was, would show me the way to picking up my sword and putting on my armor.

In the process, there would be many lessons to be learned from what went right and what had room for improvement. We wouldn't have the option to stop and pat ourselves on the back. We would have to keep pushing forward, adjusting and adapting the blueprint in response to challenges met on the ground. And there would be plenty of those.

Innovations don't always appear in the middle of the night as a brainstorm out of thin air. Luckily, one of our first steps for creating connections was something that did sort of happen that way.

If God is in the details, then the Goddess is in the connections.

—Gloria Steinem, in conversation about
the universality of rare

MAPPING AND CONNECTING RARE

In the earliest days of our foundation, I can recall hearing there might be as few as 2,000 NMO patients in the world. After getting everyone in the room and looking more closely at the data, the next guesstimate was still in the category of ultra-rare—maybe 8,000 cases worldwide.

It's tough to get a head count when many people who have NMO don't know that is what they have. No diagnosis or misdiagnosis. In fact, as we would later learn, there were different names and different treatments used for cases of NMO in other countries around the world. But the main reason it was hard to fix any real numbers was because up until we set out to cure NMO, no full-scale effort had ever been made to connect to patients.

So the question we had to figure out in the beginning had been an unexpected one. Given the logistical and privacy issues, on top of the fact that NMO sufferers were spread over large geographic distances: how were we going to find other patients?

Sure, I have always loved the idea that "if you build it, they will come." But that concept didn't hold as true as I had hoped in the early days after launching our website and starting to develop important patient resources. After more than a few sleepless nights, an idea struck one late night morning. I sat up in bed in the dark.

One of the patient resources we had already conceived was a map of the world that identified who and where the NMO experts were: *Connect the Docs*. The problem I'd been stumbling over was how we could direct patients to doctors if we couldn't locate the patients in the first place. Then I finally realized if we went ahead and developed our Connect the Docs tool, those same clinicians would connect to us, to each other, and would in turn connect their patients to us.

Why hadn't I thought of that sooner?

In no time, we set up an online map and a real one in my office and began pinpointing where we could find out about who the NMO doctors were—whether they were in the clinic or in the laboratory—and how they were diagnosing and treating patients with NMO.

To date, the Connect the Docs interactive map—which we continuously update—includes a global radar screen of as many as 300 NMO specialists from every continent except Antarctica (and we are looking for one there). This directory is now one of many tools we offer to connect patients to medical expertise as well as to us as home base.

Thinking back to those first months when so many in the patient community had been marooned alone on distant shores, I remember getting immediate responses that sounded as though we had just received an SOS for rescue from shipwreck. I understood, because we had been there ourselves.

We started hearing almost daily from physicians and medical personnel at various levels *and* soon afterward from their patients. Surprisingly— or not—many of the doctors' offices looked to us to supplement the sparse information on NMO that they had at the time or could offer to patients. Likewise, patients would frequently ask us, "Do you have any materials about NMO that I can give to my primary care doctor?" Or—"How can I inform hospital and emergency room staff about my condition?"

These were needs that had come up in planning sessions with our Advisory Board, and we were already shaping tools to help. We were developing a handbook all about NMO for patients that was comprehensive enough to give to healthcare providers. I was also working on an urgent, attention-getting bulletin to blast out to the medical community that would detail the differences between NMO and MS (and other auto-immune diseases)—a strategy to address ongoing issues of misdiagnosis, even now that there was a specific NMO blood test available. From these growing numbers of requests, I knew we would have to push harder and faster to deliver all our tools and resources to patients and doctors.

The wall map in my office was populating rapidly—NMO existed everywhere. It was simply that no one knew.

And with every email or phone call came new information that we could include in our database, all of it helping us to better map the incidence and prevalence of NMO. This was vital data needed for our cure machine.

But for me connections were never about statistics. Every aspect of each patient's story—from heartbreak to hope—mattered to me, to all of us in our NMO family. That's why whenever patients or others reached out to become part of our community or to ask for information, we responded personally and individually. I wanted to make sure they and their caregivers knew we were not merely a virtual space or press button call center. We were a home, with real people who cared and understood.

Whenever I spoke to moms and dads of NMO patients, I could relate to their anguish and the frustration of having to make fateful decisions based on almost no information. Many of those limitations, however, were starting to fall by the wayside. That much I could offer by way of reassurance.

For Bill and me, efforts to create resources to empower our NMO extended family were an outgrowth of Ali's declaration that our work to find a cure was much bigger than us alone. Whatever we learned, whatever innovative tools we developed, whatever advances in science we catalyzed—these were for the benefit of all.

This focus on how to empower every stakeholder in the journey to cure NMO and other diseases, rare or not, was embedded in my blueprint at its inception. Or as I've been known to put it: "With the power of love and intention, anything is possible."

In that spirit, I shouldn't have been surprised that out of all the Frequently Asked Questions we heard—and we sought as many answers as we could—the one that we seemed to hear from almost every patient or loved one was, "How can I help?"

That poignant question never failed to take my breath away. That was the power of some kind of rare—that those who were stricken by a terrifying and life-altering disease were asking how *they* could help.

There would be many remarkable ways that NMO patients, family members, friends, and loved ones would then take on their own roles as advocates, educators, and fund-raisers on behalf of the Foundation. After the *Spectrum* newsletter was created for the website, other patients started submitting their NMO stories. Before long, we had a permanent patient-centered blog that would replace the newsletter. We repurposed the *Spectrum* for sharing the latest research publications with the NMO patient community, the medical field at large, and with the broader public.

I think often of one mother whose daughter had initially been misdiagnosed with MS and wanted advice on how to be a more vocal advocate in getting the word out about NMO. She thought she didn't have the capacity to make a difference.

"Victoria," she confided on the phone, "I'm just a mom in Tennessee with a small voice, and you're there in Los Angeles with a big voice."

That moment confirmed one of the pillars of my blueprint—that I needed to grow all the NMO voices. Rare needed reverberation.

I reassured her that she also had a big voice, and she needed to use it. "We need your voice in Tennessee," I told her. "We need *every* voice, everywhere. This isn't the time to get quiet. This is the time to get loud."

We talked about the fact that curing a disease isn't for wimps. And certainly having a disease isn't either.

That mom from Tennessee would go on to raise her voice and to deliver NMO educational materials to medical care providers in her state and beyond. Those actions would be life-saving for others who would now benefit from a more accurate diagnosis and more appropriate treatment when symptoms of attacks first presented or relapses flared.

The bigger message was this—those who are most affected can often be the ones to have the biggest voices. And I was humbled time and again by their choice to do all they could to help end NMO.

VAMPIRE DIARIES

Whenever any patient asked how they could *most* help in making a difference, there was one answer that stood above the rest. Just short of putting
on a thick Transylvania accent, the response was, in essence, "We want to
draw your blood."

There was—and is—no way to overstate the importance of voluntary
blood donations from patients to finding answers for a rare disease. And
that is just as true for our biorepository for NMO research. Even before
our first Roundtable meeting with our researchers, we knew how limited
blood and other biospecimens would be for quantum-leap breakthroughs.
So we had already made the building of a biorepository—along with a
database for clinical data linked to those samples—an absolute priority.

In building many of the parts of the cure machine, every so often I
would have a rude awakening about an aspect we had not yet anticipated.
It would be hard not to think—*Oh, so we have to do that ourselves, too?*
In this instance, the conclusion that we would have to coordinate with
the right partners to manage our blood- and data-collection processes—
and then some—came out of a full-blown crisis for our family when a
mix-up at a lab resulted in a set of Ali's blood work being lost. Not just
any blood work. These blood draws had been collected as part of her
preparation for being treated with Rituxan (rituximab), a medication
with an informal track record for reducing the frequency of NMO relapses in some patients. Its use in NMO had just emerged as one of the
experimental treatments, repurposed from its approved use in treating B
cell lymphoma. We had also considered azathioprine—a broad-spectrum
immune suppressant that had been around the longest for use in treating
such illnesses as blood-born cancers and inflammatory bowel disease.

That was an excruciating decision, balancing known risks with possible rewards: would it be the *A* drug or the *R* drug? We reviewed all
the data we could find. There was one Mayo Clinic study, conducted by
Dr. Sean Pittock of twenty-five patients on each of the five available
treatment options, all of which included incidents of severe relapses and

death. Some of those terrifying instances had been caused by complications of NMO flare-ups, others by the side effects of the drugs themselves. After much deliberation, we opted for *R*—based on the average
reduction in relapses from three relapses a year to almost none.

Rituximab, as we learned, is a therapeutic antibody. It works by binding
to a molecule found only on the surface of B cells—which are responsible for
producing the antibody that, in NMO, mistakenly targets the AQP4 protein
water channel molecule and inflames the spinal cord, optic nerve, and brain
tissues. If you disable or delete the troublemaking B cells, that interrupts the
process that leads to inflammation and the destruction of myelin.

The science made sense. But no promises. No guarantees.

We were desperate for the benefit of preventing any relapses. At that
point, Ali had only experienced the one optical nerve attack. Aware of the
risks, we began the process of going on this regimen. This involved taking
Ali off all other medications, including daily steroids used to suppress her
immune system and stave off attacks. The purpose of the weaning off was to
be able to draw her blood before the treatment began and then compare her
baseline samples to the blood drawn after the rituximab injections—to see if
the troublemaking B cells were being cleared and if future attacks might be
prevented. Besides going off the steroids, there was yet another risk that was
constant and threatening no matter what: depleting B cells would increase
the risks of infection and cancer. The realities of those risks were cruel, although the potential benefit for no more attacks was compelling.

For the next twenty-nine days, no problems. Much to our horror,
on day thirty of tapering her off her prior medication, shortly after the
final draw of her pre-rituximab blood samples, Ali had her first transverse
myelitis attack.

The timing was a nightmare—our 2% life again. Even though Dr. Weinshenker had predicted she would probably have her first attack around that
time, I was still hoping and praying he was going to be wrong. Then, during
a family trip to New York City, Ali woke up in the middle of the night in
excruciating pain—the worst she'd felt in her life. Like knives stabbing up
and down her spine.

To make everything more surreal, her legs suddenly went numb—from her feet almost up to her waist.

We were able to get her treatment quickly—a steroid infusion that worked to alleviate the symptoms. As soon as we returned to Los Angeles, an MRI of her spinal cord confirmed we hadn't dodged the one bullet I had prayed we could.

A short time after that blow came the news that someone at the lab, not following the chain of command, had mistakenly thrown out the vials of her untreated blood. By a small stroke of luck, two extra vials of blood had been taken when Ali first visited the Mayo Clinic.

Phew. Had we at least dodged that bullet? Not so fast.

When I made the request for the vials to be transferred to the team monitoring the administration of rituximab, there were jurisdictional issues.

Serious? Yep.

After much ado, we were sent the two vials. Whether or not this ordeal colored our experience with the R drug for Ali I can't really say—although in the end, we opted to go with a different treatment regimen altogether.

The point I have to make here—for any patient of a rare or poorly understood disease where there are no approved or standard recommendations for the "drug of choice" that will produce the best outcomes for patients—you have to do your own due diligence. Work closely with your doctor to find what will be most effective and best tolerated in your case.

Out of our painstaking, maddening experience, I recognized that the Foundation needed to catalyze an analysis of treatment regimens used in NMO—drugs best used individually and in combination. That would be done by our research and advisory teams working together. And we would also want to study potential effects of these drugs on molecular and cellular biomarkers from patients themselves. To do that, of course, we would need even more blood.

Despite being in uncharted waters and having to wrap our heads around the complex logistics, our ordeal made it clear that we had to create a blood bank for NMO and a better way to manage it. Obviously, we would have to find partners in the process. It didn't take me long to learn biorepositories are strange animals. Collecting the blood or other specimens is just the first step—and one that comes with a mountain of paperwork requiring approval from institutions, researchers, and patients. But then comes processing, quality control, and storage and distribution of samples, plus the detailed policies for accessing them. We couldn't just turn over all those responsibilities without actively managing the team. Otherwise, I knew the sharing of blood for research would be an ongoing problem. We wanted a living and breathing resource for research—not a museum of unused biospecimens and data gathering permafrost in some dark warehouse. Nor did we have the luxury for errors that would result in the kind of loss of small blood samples we had just experienced.

As usual, there was pushback from the research establishment: "Why would a disease with a small patient population need its own biorepository?" "Why would you add another major task with all its moving parts to what you are already doing?"

Yet others were encouraging—especially our research clinicians and scientists at the different academic medical centers and beyond, who could now do studies they would not have been able to do otherwise.

While I had never built a blood bank, the principles were not entirely different from skill sets that both Bill and I commanded in our respective businesses: from protocol development and study site management to processing, cataloguing, archiving, and shipping—and all the quality checks and balances in between.

Blood literally was going to be the lifeblood of a cure machine.

Even though I knew how important it would be for us to make sure the process was run meticulously, I didn't yet recognize just how much this effort would crystallize my blueprint. Building an NMO biorepository, more than any other resource, would enable collaboration and accelerate lifesaving discoveries in research regarding the causes and treatment of NMO.

The second game changer that we understood about the biorepository was not intuitively obvious: The answers to solving NMO were hidden in the blood of patients *and* in their blood relatives. It was important to know what NMO was, and it was important to know what NMO *was not*. In other words, our investigators could begin to pinpoint what *caused* the disease in patients and what *prevented* the disease in unaffected family members who had very similar genetics and environmental exposures. That perspective would offer another significant key to the cure, and opportunities for everyone to help. Bottom line: the make-or-break decision by everyone invested in solving the disease would be whether they actively participated in the research or opted to watch and wait from the sideline.

And as much as joining in made sense, we would need to address the practical concerns for anyone donating their blood and medical data for research. It's a painstaking process that promises no immediate benefit other than knowing it is the rarest and most selfless act to give of yourself so that others can live.

I could never say enough about the generosity of patients and their family members who, from the start, chose to participate. From molecular causes to population effects—there was a groundswell of heroes wanting to give their blood to help find the answers.

But let's not sugarcoat the challenges. From common sense and my business knowledge of supply and demand, I saw plainly that in a rare disease like NMO, having enough blood for research was always going to be a struggle. One of the big questions right off the bat was how to get patients to the draw sites when they lived in rural locations or could not travel. Eventually, I decided, if we couldn't get those patients to the draw sites, we would bring the draw sites to them. So to speak.

MOBILE MEDICINE

Our cure machine was teaching itself to speed up time and adapt to unforeseen complications as they arose. We went low-tech when practical and high-tech when possible. We built on existing relationships and then expanded to newer ones.

Starting in 2008, and for the next four years, our blood bank was run in partnership with the Accelerated Cure Project (ACP), and in association with Dr. Ben Greenberg and his team at the University of Texas Southwestern in Dallas. For this project, UTSW served as the conduit to the researchers and helped with the process from soup to nuts. At that time, there were fifteen collection sites at different neurology clinics around the country—ten for adults and five for pediatric patients.

Even though we were piggybacking on an existing collection system, we still had to be vigilant in directing traffic and coordinating between those many draw centers. And I hadn't yet figured out how to assist patients who lived too far away from the draw centers.

Out of that frustration and challenge, an interesting solution arose in September 2009, during one of Ali's regular visits to Dr. Greenberg at UTSW. Before we headed back to Los Angeles, I had a chance to catch up with Martha Mann, a clinical research nurse who had taken on the role of NMO Repository Study Nurse for our ACP project, in charge of patient enrollment and follow-up at all the different draw sites.

I wanted to hear how the process was moving along. And because I also like to show my sincere gratitude to people helping us find cures, on that visit I came bearing gifts for her and members of the team. Just a few goody bags with some of the best-loved makeup items from my line.

As soon as we launched our foundation, I knew that the job of running my cosmetics company had to be turned over to other management. It wouldn't be the same in terms of my ability to develop new product, that's always a given. However, I had a strong team in place who could oversee the global operations for Victoria Jackson Cosmetics, still in high demand and shipping to loyal customers around the world.

Now and then, it felt good to share a bit of my former life with all the women who were in any way connected to helping cure NMO. Whether in the clinics, hospitals, offices—or in the labs working hours on end—they were giving their all to take care of NMO patients. If I could give back to remind them to take care of themselves too, even if it was just with gifts of makeup, why wouldn't I?

As we got to talking about how our repository collection process was going, I asked Martha—soft-spoken but always ready to be vocal and go the extra mile for patients—her thoughts about a new idea. I brought up the fact that I was thinking about how to reach those patients who were either hesitant to come to a draw site or who just couldn't make the trek. Martha admitted there were hurdles. For many patients who didn't feel well already, there was added anxiety in contributing blood that would not necessarily give them immediate answers about their condition. The needles alone were no fun. And yes, the toughest challenge was motivating patients and caregivers to make the trip to a sometimes-unfamiliar clinic—especially when they didn't have the means to afford travel and lodging. And then the thought of returning for any reason for future draws could be just too much for some people.

The solution, not a stretch, would be for us to somehow get medical personnel to those patients. By medical personnel, I was thinking specifically of a warm and nurturing presence like Martha, who could go on the road to enroll patients and do their blood draws in the comfort and privacy of their own homes.

Then I turned to her and asked if that was something she could do. She didn't miss a beat before saying, "Of course."

"What would you need to get going right away?" I asked, thinking about all the specialized equipment she'd require for transporting samples and getting to out-of-the-way places.

"A cooler," Martha replied. "And my car."

A traveling nurse? The idea made total sense and was in keeping with how plain and simple problem-solving is often the shortest distance between "can't" and "can."

The plan was of immediate appeal to new enrollees. And I wanted to go bigger.

How else could I add excitement and—ambitious as this may sound—*allure* to the process of contributing to the biorepository? Talking to Ali, I floated the concept of giving thank-you gifts from my makeup line to patients and family members who donated their blood and clinical data to the repository. She loved it.

Not exactly by the book, I admit. But why not? I called the program "Blush for Blood" and saw at once that it was possible to bring light and a

little color to others who'd been in the dark struggling alone with the uncertainty of a disease like NMO. It was another way to connect patients
to our community in a rare and personal way.

Ali later quipped, "Who comes up with a traveling nurse who spreads
the cheer of blush or mascara or lip gloss wherever she goes? My mom."

Over the next few years, Martha Mann's journey on the road took
her all around North America to enroll forty-six NMO patients who
would not have been able to participate in our biorepository without mo-
bile medicine—door-to-door service. To help get the word out, we sent
a videographer along with her, and I put together a short film that added
another layer of allure. In that same time frame, our Patient Days in Los
Angeles added sixty-two new enrollees—with a few draws that happened
all in one place on one day.

At first, when Ali came up with the idea for Patient Day, I don't think
the connection to being able to do blood draws even dawned on me. But
sure enough, it was a critical step in connecting to patients and expanding
the repository program. Once we connected those dots and set up the
process, it would be a real game changer for discoveries to come.

The upshot? Eventually, as the numbers in our patient community
started to grow, we could see that drawing blood from groups of patients—
like at Patient Days and other mini conferences—was the most time- and
cost-effective. Without putting all the parts together, we wouldn't have
been able to build the repository at the speed we did.

But there was still room for improvement. A big task at hand was to
do more to create standardization and consistency in biospecimen gathering. Why? Because, as I understood, when studying any disease—especially a rare one—comparing apples to apples is key. Inevitably, we would
run into challenges due to the variability of the processing and storing of
our blood samples that were taking place at the different draw sites. We
needed a system that could be accessed by scientists around the world yet
housed and organized in a more streamlined and centralized way.

Very quickly these realities led to an even more ambitious system with
new partnerships. We began working with industry giants like LabCorp

and Covance in biospecimen collection, storage, and shipment. When I was first searching for contacts in this arena, I turned to my dear friend Sherry Lansing—a blueprinter in her own right, whose Power of Rare led her to revolutionize the entertainment industry, especially for women, and who is a cofounder of Stand Up to Cancer. Sherry immediately connected me with Dr. Andy Conrad, who had great expertise in building blood banks—and he and I struck up a relationship that continued when he moved to Google/Verily later on.

In the meantime, once our biobank was set up, we reached out to Doctors Larry Cook and Michael Dean at the Data Coordination Center team at the University of Utah. They were the go-to IT experts who would oversee our clinical data repository.

The faster we were able to grow and innovate, the more I realized we couldn't just stand back and expect programs to run themselves. This was where my tendency to worry paid off—in thinking ahead about what could go right or wrong. Every blueprinter knows success can sometimes bring growing pains—and we continually had to refine our strategies.

My best advice for innovating and re-innovating is to take advantage of every resource you trust that is at your disposal—from lessons learned in the wake of crises to wisdom gained from past experiences to surrounding yourself with people who go above and beyond the call of duty.

And then sometimes the best innovations to come along are the ones you didn't plan on at all.

RIPPLE EFFECTS

Change, in my experience, doesn't happen in grand moments when rockets flare or angels sing. And it's true—the revolution doesn't always get advertised. Still, there are pivotal moments of growth that—if you pay attention—can validate all the work you've done up to that point and give you assurance that you're on the right path. I looked for the ripple effect of our work—real improvements in the lives of patients and signs that we were getting closer to big breakthroughs.

The collaborative atmosphere in the room at our 3rd Annual Round-table symposium in 2010 let me know that meaningful change had begun. For everyone present in those memorable forty-eight hours of exchange, there was a collective sense that we were about to make a quantum leap toward turning theory into practice.

Incredible as it sounds, I felt we were not just building the cure machine—we were now *flying it.*

Dr. Greenberg said as much when he recapped our discussions on Patient Day (our 2nd Annual) and told a room full of patients and care-givers, "If you compared the conversations we had these past two days with what we were talking about two years ago, they'd be *completely* different." Things that were not even on the horizon when we began, he admitted, were now being realized on a daily basis—a pace of progress he called "unparalleled anywhere in medicine." So much was changing, in fact, Dr. Greenberg noted, "We walked out of the meeting very inspired because there is real hope to make this disease a nuisance and not a problem. And someday it will be a disease that disappears."

Most hadn't anticipated coming up with answers in science and medicine so fast. After brainstorming sessions that lasted long into two nights, we had emerged with a new mechanism to unite the global expertise in NMO and fast-track the process of idea sharing and, ultimately, pave the NMO clinical trial superhighway.

We first called that mechanism the Neuromyelitis Clinical Consortium—a forerunner of the International Clinical Consortium. Including Doctors Michael Levy at Johns Hopkins, Dean Wingerchuk at the Mayo Clinic, Ben Greenberg at UTSW, and our foundation advisors, this two-year collaboration was conceived to develop *an integrated network* of centers for the advancement of NMO medical and scientific research.

Through the Consortium we established an even more defined and uniform way to go about the collection of clinical information about NMO patients. We also made it a priority—based on that information—to conduct retrospective studies of all the data collected so far. In turn, we could then prioritize new grant proposals to make sure they were laser-focused on meeting the greatest needs of patients—from diagnosis to treatments and from prevention to cures.

In two short years, many of those goals and more would be met, just in time for much more than a ripple effect but in fact a wave that would put rare on the world stage and in the spotlight.

These advances would be the result of setting even higher-bar goals: the development and validation of new diagnostic tests; evaluation of factors that might improve prevention and treatment of relapses; and, of vital importance, new ways of identifying biomarkers to decipher the severity of attacks and predict upcoming attacks.

All the while, backed by the wisdom and energy of our advisors, these advances were turned into publications in high-impact journals so that the entire world of neurology and beyond was kept up to speed. There was the international update on magnetic resonance imaging (MRI) in NMO, published in the prestigious *Journal of Neurology*. There was the state-of-the-art paper on B cells in NMO published in *Neurology: Neuroimmunology & Neuroinflammation* (known as *Neurology: NN*). There was the paper describing advanced MRI techniques in diagnosing NMO published in the high-impact Neurology division of the *Journal of the American Medical Association* (JAMA). Then, later, there would be the pivotal paper focused on challenges and opportunities in designing clinical trials for NMO published in *Neurology*—which most in the field consider to be the playbook and catalyst for the many NMO clinical trials that followed.

And our advisors would go one step further—toward cures—with the publication of two groundbreaking papers focused on the brave new science of restoring immune tolerance in NMO, published in *Neurology: NN*. Our "little foundation that could" was charging ahead, inspired, as always, by and for patients.

THE POWER OF CIRCLES

When it comes to great strategies that inspire revolutionary actions, I have had to learn—sometimes the hard way—to avoid falling in love with your own innovations. That requires a constant process of asking myself and others how we can improve what we're doing or explore and pursue a completely different pathway.

In an atmosphere of life-and-death urgency, I have had to ask myself how and when to innovate. In such instances and others, my homegrown process for decision-making can basically be divided into three parts: a) *intuition*—my trustworthy internal guidance system; 2) *adaptation*—a discipline to course-correct quickly when necessary or consider alternatives as progress evolves, even when things are going well; and 3) *manifestation*—being willing to claim accomplishments of goals when reached and use them to set even higher goals.

Most of my heavy lifting has taken place in that second stage of adaptation—when I've had to accept that a particular strategy hasn't worked—or worked so well that there would be the temptation to become complacent. We always needed to push past limits to get closer to a cure—with the awareness that goals can be more of a moving target.

Such was the case when it came time to grow the scope and influence of the Clinical Consortium. We needed to go global.

For that we would need to develop a program of such universal agreement that groups around the world would be able to find common ground. We were going to build on the work we'd already done—and enable the creation of international standards, so every researcher in the world would have equal access to the precious biospecimens and data in our biorepository.

We knew we had to start with simple steps if we wanted to own this complex process. For example, until that time only centers from the US were involved. Canada was close, and would allow our first international franchise expansion. Not rocket science—but effective. Thus the International Clinical Consortium for NMO was born.

Originally our goal for the International Clinical Consortium (ICC) was dubbed "12 by 12." That is, we wanted to recruit twelve of the most renowned centers in the world to lead the charge for solving NMO with us, and to have these sites up and running by the end of 2012. Within months, we doubled our target numbers in recruiting the most visionary and passionate clinicians from around the world to be part of ICC. We were connecting leading minds around the world to focus on a rare disease, and soon the ICC would become among the largest international research collaboratives on any autoimmune disease, let alone any rare disease. Today there are nearly 80 of the absolute best and brightest experts in the world in the ICC.

At the same time, our other brainchild—CIRCLES—would do what only my imagination could once conceive possible.

The program came out of the deepening challenge we faced making optimal use of our growing biorepository. CIRCLES—which stands for Collaborative International Research in Clinical and Longitudinal Experience Study—would be a first of its kind. Calling this natural history of a rare disease a complex undertaking was a kind way to break the news to the faint of heart. Even so, by collecting consistent clinical information and biospecimens at every site, we would make sure that every drop of blood and bit of data would yield the most meaningful results. And all the findings would be accessible to everyone.

When I first heard what we were going to be studying and how much was to be learned, I was amazed. But I admit to wondering, *What do they mean by longitudinal?* Was this something about latitude and longitude? Was there a map in all this? And what was a natural history? I soon learned that natural history referred to monitoring the course of a disease over time. CIRCLES was both observational and longitudinal in that patients and comparative volunteers would be followed over time—to observe the natural history of their particular case in relation to others. In this longitudinal study, we could track the course of NMO disease in patients on a consensus-based, apples-to-apples comparison that connected multiple investigational sites.

CIRCLES would reach beyond the study of NMO patients to also include the biospecimens from patients with other autoimmune diseases. CIRCLES would also make it possible, more than ever, to study the biospecimens we collected from patients' blood relatives who did not have

NMO—whose genetic similarities to patients served as controls. This was where we'd really be able to home in on not just what was going *wrong* in the molecular mechanisms of NMO patients—but also what was going *right* with family members and others whose immune systems were healthy.

It's worth repeating that this kind of rare thinking was the catalytic force that changed the treatment of HIV/AIDS—from thirty pills a day (with horrific side effects) to just one pill a day, which keeps most patients symptom-free. Dr. Yeaman—an infectious diseases specialist by day—reminded us how that happened: because a few rare researchers thought to study why individuals who might have been exposed to HIV somehow didn't contract the virus.

With that kind of approach, CIRCLES studies would lead to a series of unprecedented insights about the immune system—with major implications that went beyond NMO. As Dr. Yeaman put it: "NMO lets us see through the keyhole into a new room that has never been seen before."

Now that is the Power of Rare.

As these facets of our new program were being realized, I remembered a conversation I had with Gloria Steinem—who is not only one of my personal role models but who happens to have become a dear friend over the years. It was Gloria who pointed out that part of my revolution was about creating circles rather than hierarchies in the medical space. Circles have also been a theme in the women's movement. In fact, articulating the values and actions for taking on the status quo actually began in women's conversation circles. From collaboration to courage and ultimately to change.

Though there were differences, no doubt, I could see that our CIRCLES studies were quickly becoming bigger than what we first envisioned.

When we began CIRCLES, we started with four sites that were each headed by investigators who had distinguished themselves, through peer recognition, as leaders in the field. Today there are fifteen sites in the United States and one in Canada—and counting. And, even more astounding, we will soon exceed 1,000 patients who have signed up to be part of CIRCLES—two years ahead of schedule for the target we had boldly set.

No more hitting the road for Martha and her cooler.

This isn't to say there weren't growing pains. With the success of this rapid expansion of a cutting-edge biomedical operation came new challenges. In turn, we would have to rev the engines of the cure machine to innovate. As it turned out, to do the most modern research in NMO, researchers needed the most modern reagents. For example, to study how T or B cells respond incorrectly to the AQP4 protein, we would need to contract the manufacturing of the highest-quality AQP4 protein reagent for research. Likewise, to investigate the molecular mechanisms of NMO-IgG antibody—yep, we would need to pay for production of that as well. Of course, the many reagents and resources generated would all be made available to researchers around the world, and free of charge. Because we had committed to funding research from the start, we had to reduce the barriers to breakthroughs, and so we did.

Hmmm. Somehow I'd gone from producing lip gloss and mascara, to recombinant human AQP4 protein and engineered NMO-IgG antibody.

As always, patients and their families chose to give back in a beautiful circle of gratitude as well. The NMO patient community, more and more, adopted the attitude that every time they participated in a study and every time they made a contribution to the biorepository, it was an act of altruism for themselves, for one another, and for millions of other patients with autoimmune diseases, both rare and common.

I remember that point being made forcefully during a Patient Day Q&A by Janis—one of the first of our NMO family I met early on—who believed very passionately in educating the public and fellow patients about the latest findings in our research. What Janis said, in urging others to participate in clinical studies, was, "If it benefits you, then it will benefit all of us—and vice versa."

Later, I pulled her aside and thanked her for her strength. It was contagious.

As important as it has been to give patients open access to information from our investigators, it's just as important that researchers—be they clinical, translational, or basic science—have access to feedback from patients. From telling symptoms to treatment side effects, and from quality of life to fears and concerns, every story counts.

Educating and communicating with one another—connecting all the parts of our growing global community—would be an ongoing process. So too was the major undertaking of starting to educate the medical community and the public at large. Educating one another truly can be saving each other.

> # I find it inspiring and humbling to meet NMO patients who are participating in research studies. This represents an amazing degree of commitment, optimism, and trust, and is a truly motivating experience.
>
> —Gerald T. Nepom, MD, PhD
> *Director, Immune Tolerance Network,*
> *Benaroya Research Institute, Seattle*

KNOW MORE NMO

Ask anyone who knows me well, and they will tell you I am not one to linger in the past or rehash what happened yesterday. That is both my nature and a choice I make out of necessity—to keep my focus steeled on what must be done today and tomorrow and all the days to come—so that all the members of our NMO patient family have the best chance to live healthier, happier, and better lives.

At the same time, it's been impossible to avoid recalling that period when NMO first came into our family and how little was known about it. When we started learning the extent to which so many in our patient community had originally been misdiagnosed with MS or other conditions, like Sjogren's syndrome, lupus, "unexplained" optic neuritis, and transverse myelitis—often with waits leading to tragic consequences—I was adamant that we take bold action to demand the immediate attention of the medical establishment. My fervent intention was that no patient would ever again have to wait months or years for a correct diagnosis—of NMO or other autoimmune diseases.

A number of interesting electronic bulletin strategies were suggested, but none of them hit the mark. That was until I realized there was nothing wrong with doing something old-school now and then. Back to the chalkboard. Why couldn't we develop a way to message the fact that NMO IS NOT MS in the space of a simple pamphlet—the kind you see in many doctors' offices—but designed in the most eye-catching, colorful manner with wording that could not be ignored?

And that's what we did. In hopeful green hues, the brochure had both "NMO" and "MS" in compelling graphics to invite curiosity from anyone who happened to glance at it. In clean, direct language, the copy inside made it clear: "What Is NMO?" In relatable terms, the writing went on to summarize how NMO, MS, and some other autoimmune disease *symptoms* were alike—but that the diseases were very different. The brochure also compared the current diagnostic criteria and how treatments for the different diseases were different. The content was intended to be eye-opening too:

Until recently, Neuromyelitis Optica was thought to be a type of Multiple Sclerosis. However, recent discoveries indicate that NMO and MS are distinct diseases. Traditionally spinal cord lesions seen in NMO are longer than MS but this is not always the case. With so many symptoms in common, NMO can sometimes be confused with MS or other diseases. But these diseases are treated in different ways and early detection and treatment help ensure best outcomes.

Similar Symptoms

NMO symptoms can vary from person to person and may re-
semble MS symptoms in many ways. NMO is most commonly
characterized by inflammation of the spinal cord/or optic nerves,
causing any of the following symptoms:

• Rapid onset of eye pain or loss of vision (optic neuritis).
• Limb weakness, numbness, or paralysis (transverse myelitis).
• Shooting pain or tingling in the neck, back, or abdomen.
• Loss of bowel and bladder control.
• Prolonged nausea, vomiting, or hiccups.

Sometimes these symptoms are temporary, and resolve on their
own. In any case, it is important to discuss these symptoms with
your doctor to help consider NMO in your diagnosis.

NMO-IgG Antibody Test

The recent discovery of an antibody in the blood of individuals with NMO gives doctors a reliable biomarker to distinguish
NMO from MS. The antibody, known as NMO-IgG, seems to
be present in about 70 percent of those with NMO and is not
found in people with MS or other similar conditions. The test can
be ordered by any primary care physician.

We provided contact information for reaching out to the Foundation,
plus a list of resources to request from us, and other suggestions.

In 2011, the estimated number of NMO cases had grown to 35,000.
So symbolically our first printing was 35,000 copies of the brochure—but
we wanted more than just patients to know NMO. We targeted the offices
of neurologists and ophthalmologists, as well as emergency room doctors
and several other locations where, we had learned from previously misdiagnosed patients, NMO might not typically be familiar to personnel.

Today, that original brochure, updated frequently into multiple re-
printings, has been translated into more than ten languages and distrib-
uted globally. For many medical providers and patients alike, the "Little
Brochure That Could" has provided life-saving information.

NMO may not yet be a household name—although you can bet I'm
working on that—but there is most encouraging news to report. At our
latest Patient Day, I learned that on average a delayed diagnosis time is
only three weeks for newly symptomatic NMO patients. For many, once
the blood test is sent in, the wait can be as short as four or five days. And
the accuracy of diagnosis has dramatically improved as well—meaning
patients are receiving the best care as quickly as possible.

But we still have a long way to go.

Even so, I'm heartened to witness over and over again evidence that
empowered and informed patients are unstoppable. More and more, we
started hearing patients quoting recent research results and asking questions that were as insightful than any doctor's questions in the room. They
keep all of us on our toes. And they keep us all moving forward.

If knowledge is power—and there is no doubt about that—empowerment
happens when a space is created for every question, no matter how seemingly
insignificant. Unfortunately, the modern healthcare system really does not
offer the time or capacity to fully educate patients—especially when it comes
to a rare disease that even most clinicians know little about. And that's why
we desperately need a revolution that empowers patients with knowledge
and options and doesn't leave them feeling overwhelmed. Even for those
who don't have a rare condition, there are more challenges than ever in inter-
acting with medical personnel or insurance offices, in processing the daunting amounts of paperwork and bills, and in all the real and perceived barriers
to patient care.

Born of my own fear-based questions and all the questions from our
patient community—an idea for our own NMO bible was presented to
me by our advisors. My first question was, how fast could we get it done?
A team was assembled from among our dedicated thought leaders to get
it written, and they leapt into action. My focus was on selecting every

photograph and design element to make every page as uplifting and empowering—and not scary—as I could.

Before long, we had completed the first edition of the *NMO Patient
Resource Guide: What You Need to Know*. Its purpose is stated right after
the title page:

> This guide may be a companion, a mentor, a compass, a friend –
> all meant to support you on your journey with NMO. Whether
> you are a patient, a caregiver, or someone who just wants to learn
> more about NMO, we hope that you can find some answers to
> unanswered questions, a helping hand where there was no help,
> or perhaps a sympathetic ear as you gain comfort and knowledge
> from the resources in this guide and in the Foundation's online
> community. Because this book offers a great deal of informa-
> tion, we encourage you to pace yourself. In navigating the world
> of NMO, we hope this guide may serve as an interactive tool in
> which you can take notes, highlight text, keep a diary, write down
> more questions or ideas, and anything else you think will help you
> live with NMO.
>
> You may have NMO—*but NMO does not have you.*

The guide is now in its third edition—with a reach of more than 25,000
readers to date. I know of no other resource of its kind and scope ever developed for a rare disease population. Even compared to materials available
for more common diseases, our guide is rarer still as a handbook for NMO
patients—and for their selfless caregivers and support systems—plus their
healthcare providers, whose knowledge of NMO has often been limited.

For patients, their families, and caregivers, this guide is our reference
point—with main subject tabs that include: NMO Explained, History
& Discovery, Treatment & Management of NMO, Living with NMO
(covering everything that affects the quality of life for every patient and
caretaker), and an extensive section on NMO science breakthroughs
called Hope for the Future. At the back of the hard copy notebook and

digital versions (downloadable from our app or website), there are sections called Resources & Support, Directory of Clinicians (our Connect the Docs), and Glossary of Key Terms & Facts.

A handy one-stop shop for information on all things NMO? Absolutely. Again, many of these resources have come about because I also wanted to create a sense of belonging and connection that had been lacking for us when Ali was first diagnosed. And so it has been enormously heartwarming to experience what I have heard from so many in our NMO community—"Thank you for letting us know that we are not alone."

Whether we meet in person, in the pages of our Patient Guide, online, or in the growing number of support groups that are emerging around the world, I believe that all of us feel the tremendous groundswell that is happening around NMO. From all corners of the globe, our advocacy community is making its voice known.

In our blueprint, we began with two options: a) accept the status quo; or b) choose to be bold. We went for bold. But the key for me was never to rest on our laurels once interim goals were achieved. So we went for bolder still—*How could we push higher and get there faster?*

Even so, sometimes I had to be reminded how far we had come in a short amount of time. Jacinta Behne—who directs the operations team at the offices of the Guthy-Jackson Charitable Foundation and whose curriculum vitae includes having worked for NASA (keeping rocket ships running on schedule and the like, no big deal)—once compared our progress on NMO in just a few years to us having gone from horse and buggy to the moon buggy. And she would know.

I know the early progress wouldn't have happened without true collaboration among all stakeholders in our NMO community. This was the heartbeat of our blueprint. With everyone from around the world being in the same place at the same time, focused on the same goal, something transformational happens. It does take a village. It takes problem solvers who recognize the real challenges—from patient insiders living with a rare autoimmune disease and from outsiders who bring new thinking to make a difference. *Inside-out* and *outside-in* solutions to NMO.

RARE DAYS FOR RARE PATIENTS

When you choose to face fear in the battle to unmask a devastating disease like NMO, I also believe you are entitled to a timeout or two to vent. These are well deserved, moments to throw down as much ranting, railing, or irreverent humor as you can muster. Mostly I try to choose the latter, and I am known for floating slogans and whatnot by Ali, like, "Well, instead of 'Stand Up to Cancer!' maybe we should have 'Jump Up Really High for NMO!'"

Once, she made me promise that when we found the cure to NMO, and if it were a therapeutic antibody, we would call it the Alibody

Ali also had a high tolerance for some of my more radical ideas for innovations—*except* when they had the potential to veer into the realm of faith healing or even snake oil buying. Yes, it's true, occasionally, in my desperation to be open to alternative modalities, I would entertain novel treatments that weren't just rare but that frankly went against my better judgment. I seem to recall a psychic who charged a lot of money for a juicing remedy. And then there was the spiritualist who had cured autoimmune diseases—in canine populations.

I was open to all possibilities, but there were lessons learned from this process. Sometimes the best-intentioned actions did send me in wrong directions—smack into dead ends or off on a detour when seeking advice from sellers disguising pseudoscience as miracle remedies. The desperate mother fueled by hope can be a vulnerable target. The old adage applied: when it sounds too miraculous to be true, it usually is. In such cases, as I'd often remind myself, let your intuition be your guide.

At the same time, as Ali might be the first to remind me, sometimes valuable innovations do come out of that same openness to outsider approaches and rare thinking. In fact, every year when planning for our Roundtable and Patient Day conferences, I would always look to bring in a few new and provocative voices to expand our imagination.

At each successive conference, the Foundation team and I really do push the limit, pulling out all the stops to keep the three days absolutely fresh, exciting, relevant, and rare. But that means the bar goes from high to higher and higher. For the Roundtable keynote lectures, I usually bring in speakers or experts who come from far outside the world of NMO but who can prod and challenge the thinking of all the NMO stakeholders, so they leave far more fired up than when they arrived. We create an inviting yet stimulating ambience for enhancing their collective brainpower. I will go to many lengths to make sure the ballrooms look less like a familiar conference setting and more like festive gatherings that nobody would want to miss. Every now and then, smoke and mirrors can make all the difference in cultivating that very setting in which big, bold, and break-through ideas begin to click.

Similarly, from the moment when patients and their family members or caretakers begin to arrive at the hotel, I want them to feel that they have left behind some of their burdens and challenges. Many of these are discussed in detail in our Patient Guide section on *Living with NMO*— and I urge anyone passionate about patient care to peruse those pages and consider how a medical revolution must address quality-of-life concerns in all patient populations. A sampling of the chapter subheadings that address challenges for NMO patients includes: *Fitness, Managing Fatigue, Coping with Vision Loss, Managing Bowel and Bladder Problems, Occupational Therapy, Support with Daily Life, Daily Living Equipment, Modifying Your Home, Driving and Transportation, Social Security Disability Benefits in the US, and Support for Caregivers.*

Many of those issues are ones I address each year by inviting outside expertise in our afternoon breakout sessions on Patient Day. Sometimes I might want to share something new and exciting that I've recently discovered—Transcendental Meditation, therapeutic writing, and so on. We have half-hour blocks of time and rotate from room to room so patients and their companions can attend as many as possible. Session topics we've offered include: Managing Stress & Fatigue, Nutrition & Diet, Pain Management, NMO in the Workplace, Simplifying the Science of NMO, Everything You Wanted to Know but Were Afraid to Ask, Bowel & Bladder Management, Sexual Dysfunction, Patients' Rights,

Complementary Medicine, Future Therapeutics, Pregnancy & NMO, Healthcare & Insurance, Pediatric NMO, Recognizing & Treating Attacks, Caretakers' Self-Care, and the all-time most-attended, Ask the Docs, which gives patients in small groups the freedom to ask doctors questions they might not in the larger morning session.

Patient Day is, for all intents and purposes, the holiest day of the year for our foundation. And as much as we honor and are forever grateful to NMO medical pioneers, patients are why we persevere.

Every year, as patients and companions unite, we try to add new touches—a social hour for reconnections and new introductions, an organizational meeting for regional advocacy groups to meet, and, as a step up from Blush for Blood, afternoon beauty makeovers and swag bags filled with the best makeup around. After we offered them the first time, the makeovers were such a hit that we have included them almost every year since.

And why not?

For more than twenty years, I had recruited fellow makeup artists to volunteer with me to do makeovers at programs I developed for women in hospitals and shelters, as well as for women in prison. And now those same dear friends and volunteers show up every year on the eve and morning of Patient Day to do makeovers for the women of our NMO community. The reactions are heartfelt, joyous, and poignant. The truth still holds—when you look better, you feel better. And when you feel better, you can change the world and help achieve a cure for NMO.

We even turn the blood draw room into a place of welcome. This is where many family members, as well as patients, donate to the program for the first time. The atmosphere is charged with the energy of positivity and possibility. The last thing we want it to look like is some antiseptic hospital setting. We set up a buffet of snacks and beverages, with colorful flowers at every draw table, and fly in the familiar smiling faces from many of our CIRCLES draw centers—who already know some of the patients and are eager to do follow-ups.

Every year, I listen for themes that come from those in attendance, making mental notes for strategies and actions to continue to adapt and manifest. At the same time, I have to allow myself to appreciate a building buzz of optimism and, well, pride in our collective courage and dedication to one another.

Somehow this cure machine has unified us in our shared revolution from within.

The greatest resource of the GJCF is community. While many research organizations promote collaboration, the GJCF has fostered an NMO research community where basic scientists, clinicians, allied health personnel, and patients have come together to work towards a common goal of curing a devastating disease. The synergism is evident in the immense progress to date and the impact that NMO research has had on patient care and our understanding of other autoimmune disorders.

—Jeffrey L. Bennett, MD, PhD

ON BECOMING A GLOBAL FAMILY

Part of the shock of being an NMO parent comes from recalling that when you bring a life into the world, your whole being is devoted to giving—not saving—your child's life. And I think about that every time I meet a parent whose daughter or son has received her or his own diagnosis out of the blue. We all know the feeling of having joined a club we didn't sign up for. We would give anything to trade places with our daughter or son, or have history choose another deal of the cards. Yet that does not and cannot happen, and dwelling on such fantasy is wasted energy we need to create change for our loved ones and for one another. So we cling to the strength that exists in not having to go it alone—in our extended family.

What is it that binds all of us together?

The word that comes most to mind—and one I keep close to my heart as essential to my understanding of the Power of Rare—is *resilience*. Sometimes that capacity even borders on *transcendence*. Or such are the feelings inspired in me whenever we come together as a community—when I take a moment to appreciate our transformation.

In the historical equivalent of the blink of an eye, a cure machine had been built to solve NMO and was readying for a movement to carry it forward. We had realized goals that others had once questioned could be achieved, and quickly. We were seeing the difference in the quality of life for patients and their caregivers—with more rapid and accurate diagnoses, earlier and more appropriate treatments, less extreme relapses or disabilities, and amazingly improved prognoses.

It's not that we hadn't experienced sorrow in our NMO family. I had come to know of too many lives that were lost. One is too many. There is no other way to confront the reality of this disease than to acknowledge how tragic its dimensions can be—which makes our work even more necessary, even more urgent. The question I could never escape was always rearing its ugly head: *Why?*

Why does this disease or any disease rob us of our babies? Or of our sisters, parents, brothers, friends, spouses, neighbors, or coworkers? Why can't we please, please charge up a revolution in caring so that we can harness the solutions that already exist and do more to end the suffering?

We, as a global community, have to continue to voice that question to the world and then increasingly take action. That's an absolute tenet of our blueprint.

It is what I mean by saying that taking on the status quo is not for the faint of heart.

A short time ago, as I sat in the back of our largest-ever hotel ballroom during our Power of Rare Patient Day, I listened as a young man stood up to ask a question of one of the clinicians about the current treatment options for NMO. This young man began his question by saying, "*We* were diagnosed less than a year ago . . ."

He glanced down at the young woman who sat next to him and lovingly placed his hand on her shoulder.

My first thought was—*How could it be possible that the two of them were each diagnosed at the same time?* That was when one of the doctors on the panel gently asked, "Now, do *you* have NMO?"

The young man was quick to explain that he was there with his wife, who was the NMO patient. Even as he made that distinction clear, I watched many in the room nod their heads in understanding. And some, like me, had to blink back the tears.

Of course. For anyone who cares deeply for the person who has NMO, the diagnosis also applies. How could it be otherwise? This was yet another reminder of what we have known from the start—that a "rare" disease is not at all rare when it affects you or someone you love.

He was making a statement about all of us—our NMO family. Without question, the era of being alone in the dreaded dark wilderness of a mystery diagnosis is no more. We have become a "we," and the connections that have been forged have made it so. We triumph when advances achieved together bring news that members of our community are doing much better. We suffer one another's pain and struggles with NMO—and we grieve for each loss.

Hope is our superpower—the essence of resilience and transcendence in the face of true challenge. We don't have the luxury of falling into despair. We must act. We know that lives can be saved and the worst damage prevented if the right treatment can be given when attacks first strike. We have a solemn duty to grow awareness at every turn. We can do that, and we must.

With whatever revolutionary and other means possible.

The simplest and most universal lessons of all came out of those early years of laying down the Foundation—no pun intended—of our blueprint. Getting started on any endeavor is tough, but the real tests come when you've left behind any signs of familiarity. So call these a blueprinter's survival kit for not giving up once you've left sight of the shore:

- Savor the good days and endure the bad days. Deal with them—preferably one at a time.

- Shift into the gear that brings you hope. Yes, there will be setbacks, plenty of them. Move forward anyway. Remember to adapt, innovate, and reinvent.

- Let the problem-solving capacities in your DNA serve as preparation for unforeseen pitfalls. You have what you need to rise above the challenges—or work around them.

- There will be critics and doubters. Smile and invite them to join the mission.

- There will be egos and tempers and battles for credit over turf. Use that energy to build a better cure machine—or shake them loose when you must. No one drama king or queen can mute the wisdom of the crowd.

- There will be charlatans—thank them for their opinion and move on.

- There will be costs—time, money, and more. Find a way.
- There will be tears. Let them fall freely. They will keep the journey real.

Realist though I have to be, I look back to our formative years with daily inspiration and overwhelming gratitude for every person who chose to walk this road with us—everyone who made possible truly great days filled with small victories and global triumphs. There were breakthroughs when none seemed possible. There were unexpected kindnesses and acts of sacrifice that melted hearts and barriers. There were moments of truth that replaced suffering and misfortune with healing and hope. There were connections and families, and bonds made and renewed and strengthened. And yes—as important as any of these—there were lives saved and lives improved on this improbable journey traveled in our one-of-a-kind cure machine. All in preparation to engage others who had never before considered the Power of Rare.

We do not need magic to change the world, we carry all the power we need inside ourselves already: we have the power to imagine better.

—J.K. Rowling

CHAPTER 5

MARKETING, MONEY, MOLECULES, AND MIRACLES

"Mom on a Mission? Yeah, we've covered a lot of those stories. What else do you have?"

A TV producer said this to me matter-of-factly early in our NMO journey. She asked this question just after I finished telling her our deeply emotional story and why I was trying desperately to raise the volume on a rare "orphan" disease.

I pressed on—hopeful that if I made the connection between NMO and the growing global threat of an autoimmune epidemic, she might reconsider.

Nope. She dismissed me, explaining how most media outlets were already overly saturated with stories that pulled at the heartstrings. Besides, she went on, getting buy-in from network and advertising execs about an issue that did not, on the surface, have big, sexy numbers was too much of a risk.

Were her comments the worst I heard? Unfortunately not. Callous as such attitudes might seem, they weren't uncommon—and I couldn't just ignore them. There was a measure of reality in her words. As a media and marketing veteran, that much I knew—just as I knew we would have to find a way to put the little disease that could on the global map. We were going to have to tell its story to the world and make it relatable to people who didn't necessarily understand science. We had to find a way to make a rare disease personal—to everyone.

First, however, we had to get past the gatekeepers of many locked doors.

I have a switch somewhere inside me—a survival instinct—that when flipped on helps me turn frustration and even despair into action. It comes through with a voice that urges me to find an alternative route and not give up. If I couldn't get in the door, then I'd get in through the window. If I couldn't get in the window, then I'd come up through the floor or down from the ceiling. And that's exactly what happened.

By 2012—just four years in—we'd created enough momentum to bring NMO out of the shadows and onto center stage of many forms of media. How was that possible? I have to give some credit to the rejection faced in the early going. As I see it, rejection can be a *Stop* sign or a *Go* sign. I chose to see it as the latter, and that definitely brought out the fighter and creative thinker in me.

Obviously, we had a marketing problem, and we had to fix it.

In the medical space, the need for marketing tends to be an afterthought or even a practice that some suggest takes away from the nobility of curing diseases and saving lives. Yet I would argue that you can't achieve cures without marketing. We needed to make our case to overcome apathy and the mind-set that a rare disease like NMO was fate and that nothing could be done about it. Too low on the priority list. We needed to build a global audience that cared. We needed a workaround to show them why they should care.

Marketing mattered. It connected to every aspect of our mission—from the molecules we were identifying in our research to turning those molecules into new therapies and ultimately creating miracles in the lives of NMO patients and their families. We had to make the best use of every penny we had invested in our mission. *Marketing, money, molecules, and miracles*—those four *M*s kept me busy.

Our messaging—yes, another *M*—had to be innovative and bold. We had an important story to tell and a responsibility to tell it—to save and improve lives and to change the world for the better.

Even when the real challenges of living with NMO and the other autoimmune diseases were troubling and not always positive, we had to find a way to be real *and* uplifting. For one thing, media consumers in the age of the Internet were savvier and more discerning. And for another, patients deserved to be represented truthfully. Even with the promising research breakthroughs, we had all the more reason to avoid the pitfalls of peddling false hopes. Besides, as every great marketer knows, ultimately there is nothing more compelling than a true story.

The bottom line? Our storytelling had to be honest and authentic.

THE HEALING POWER OF STORIES

Many of the strategies needed for getting the word out about rare had actually been percolating in me for years. For much of my life before NMO, my passion had been volunteering and working with women in jails, shelters, and hospitals. Through the vehicle of makeup and the empowerment programs I developed for those settings, I had the privilege of helping give voice to those whose stories rarely got told. And thanks to the success of my media platform in the universe of beauty, I had gone on to produce filmed stories of rarity and heroism—profiles I believed audiences would embrace if given the chance. And they did.

What I learned in the process was that the power of storytelling comes down to that open place in each of our hearts and minds that says, *Wow, if that person can confront and overcome big challenges and heal in some way, then I can too.*

By creating a space for discoveries about the self, I witnessed first-hand that just as beauty and revolution both must come from within, so too does the journey toward healing. Something miraculous and profound happens when we are able to shift how we see ourselves, the world, and others. That brings us back to "know thyself." As I had learned, knowing thyself is one of the most important abilities encoded into healthy cells and molecules of our immune systems—or autoimmune diseases, if things go wrong. It's also an important element of storytelling.

The message from the storyteller to the listener then becomes universal: we're *all* rare and yet we're all connected by common bonds. That truth, learned from experience, was woven into our global marketing plan, and would help to bring NMO out of the shadows.

> Although setbacks of all kinds may discourage us, the grand old process of storytelling puts us in touch with strengths we may have forgotten, with wisdom that has faded or disappeared, and with hopes that have fallen into darkness.

> —Nancy Mellon
> *Author, Storytelling and the Art of Imagination*

GIVING VOICE TO RARE

I've probably always been an activist for bringing untold stories to light and—no surprise—for going against the traditional marketing grain. As a communicator, I've always looked for an opening to connect my personal story to those of others, no matter how different our lives. My wish to empower anyone else in struggle comes from having walked in similar shoes. If I could overcome a challenging childhood and adolescence to become a self-made success—without any formal education or economic support—

that was proof that others could too. The message "If I can do this, so can you" was partly what motivated me to teach a college-level visual arts course called Makeup for Photography at UCLA. Even though my career was starting to take off as an in-demand makeup artist working with the world's top photographers and celebrities, I still worried that no one would sign up. Lo and behold, the classroom was filled every term I taught the course.

The class wasn't to talk about my career fortunes or hold myself up as some kind of guru. Rather, my goal was to empower my students to stop giving so much power to beauty experts of the time—and to encourage makeup artists to trust their own sensibilities in bringing out the rare beauty in every person. To take the pressure off, I'd say, "Look, it's not like we're curing cancer or anything."

Flash-forward: What were the odds that I would one day take on the role of curing a life-threatening disease? Pretty rare, I'd say. Maybe 2%.

In teaching, I turned the tables on the traditional beauty aesthetic of the late 1980s and early 1990s—a masklike foundation that sat on top of the skin and was overly tinted with oranges and other colors not always known to the natural world. Going against the status quo resulted in a pretty successful run for my class for nearly two decades. But more important, it also marked a new era in beauty aesthetics that the next generation of makeup artists who studied with me would adopt in their careers. All of this went against cookie-cutter or one-size-fits-all makeup. We were celebrating the innate beauty in each woman as unique only to her.

Own your rare.

Everything I taught and learned about seeing the beauty in rare—in ourselves, in others, and in the world—was reinforced in my more than twenty-five years of working as a volunteer with women and girls in shelters, hospitals, and jails.

So much so that when infomercial fame led to a role as a TV correspondent doing the traditional beauty beat for ABC's *The Home Show*, those were the rarely told stories I wanted to find a way to tell.

Going out on a limb, I pitched the producers the idea of filming makeovers in some of the settings where I'd been volunteering.

"Beauty—in a jail or shelter?" asked one of the producers.

"Yes."

"How would that work?"

All I could do was speak from the heart about my experiences—about the program I developed in my very early days for the Children of the Night project to stop child sex trafficking. It was the story about my working with girls who had been prostitutes or had been exploited in the sex trade—helping them to realize they didn't have to wear all that war paint.

"War paint?" the producers asked.

This conversation echoed in my memory when I first faced the challenges of connecting NMO to a broader audience. There is something universal about the discovery of self on the inside that applies as much to the immune system as it does to the expression of appearance on the outside.

For a girl or a woman on the street, war paint is an extreme use of makeup that's put on to shield her from the realities of the work—an adaptation to minimize the toll of emotionless relationships. Changing the outside, as these women transitioned to new lives, helped give them a new sense of identity.

The truth is that patients often have to wear a different kind of war paint, a mask that hides their pain and struggle for health from the world. Knowing that life and health are not just how the world sees us—but rather, more important, how we see ourselves—I always looked for ways to help others see the beauty and resilience below the surface.

Learning how to tell the stories of those who were able to see their own rare beauty and have healthier perceptions of themselves gave me a fundamental understanding of the identity crisis that goes on in autoimmunity. And the experience also informed my marketing strategies for helping make NMO relevant and personal to outsiders.

During my pitch to *The Home Show* producers, I didn't have the same grasp on the connections to rare, but I did know it was wrong for any of us to judge the conditions that created the struggles. Everyone is going through something. Our stories are what connect us to each other.

When a person is diagnosed with any disease—especially a rare and life-threatening one—everything she knows or believes about herself is brought into question. This was evident in the workshops I led for women in cancer clinics. It wasn't enough that these women suffered from cancer. For most of them, radiation and chemotherapy caused hair loss, fatigue, and depression—robbing them of their basic identity. In simple ways, makeup was the means for me to help them reclaim themselves or to take back some control—whether it was showing them how to create eyebrows when they had lost theirs or more spiritually helping them see their real beauty had not been lost. In return, I was empowered by their strength and fearlessness. Being closer to death, they said, made them closer to life. Those were the rarely expressed understandings that brought me to tears every time. In them was a message of faith that I believed audiences needed too.

What really got the attention of the producers at *The Home Show* was how I described going to jail for twenty years.

"Wait, you went to jail?"

"Of course," I replied. Or words to that effect.

Then I recounted how I worked with incarcerated women in the catacombs of the Los Angeles Twin Towers Correctional Facility. And that was despite the acute claustrophobia I had to overcome to get down there. Why did I keep going back? Because if there was a way to change how the women behind bars saw themselves and saw the world, it was a gift to me to try and make a difference in their lives—their futures.

Makeovers were always more than just about makeup.

As I told the producers, talking about how to use the mascara wand or how to apply lip gloss—these were only jumping-off points for the women to start to imagine who they wanted to be once they were released. The conversation might have been about lashes and lips, but the point was about something much bigger—again, how they saw themselves and how they felt about the way others saw them.

Many of the women in jail had been turned into warriors because of gangs and turf wars—making for tension inside the jail too.

Every time I went in, I would speak to that, asking, "For the next two hours, I want you to just park all that aside. Any problems with that?"

No one objected. Then I handed out makeup bags, and it seemed even the most hardened inmates became girls again, no longer in battle mode. I remember one of the toughest gals in there putting on her makeup and turning to another from a rival gang—and just asking, "Does this look good?" All of a sudden, it was a different room.

Many of these women were used to covering their eyebrows with foundation and drawing in thin, angular eyebrows higher up on their foreheads. Like warrior masks.

One middle-aged woman protested that she didn't want to let go of the old look that made her feel fierce.

"Okay," I said. "But can you tell me what you think your makeup should say to the world about you?"

She looked at herself in the mirror after applying her makeup as she always had. Then she shrugged and said, "Pull over?"

Everyone cracked up. "Pull over" appeal—flagging down a man who might be attracted to that look—could never be denied. Even so, once she blended her newfound foundation, she chose a more pastel palette of colors and softened her lines to reveal her authentic eyebrows. I saw her transform at the sight of herself in the mirror.

"What do you think you say to the world now?" I asked.

"That I'm a lady."

My argument to the producers was that the ability to inspire others to see themselves differently and to see life differently had been powerful for me, and I knew there was an audience out there that would respond emotionally to those moments too.

Most of the time when you pitch an idea that has never been tried before, media gatekeepers will say no because it's never been tried before or there's no proof it will work. However, when you can make them laugh or cry or feel empathy—that can change their minds and get them to care. That's what happened with *The Home Show* producers. Suddenly, rare mattered to them.

The same was true, as I'd found, for doctors and scientists and other analytical problem solvers when first encountering a rare challenge.

And so, after much deliberation, I was given the green light to film and anchor segments we shot in hospital settings and in programs for women beginning new lives, and even in the Twin Towers of the L.A. jail system. Nothing like it was being shown on television at the time. Attention for these segments went through the roof.

After that, the producers gave me carte blanche to film makeover stories of individual women who had overcome adversity. One of them I will never forget was a mother raising a son with a rare disease—who was so grateful to be able to gain some attention for his illness by appearing in our segment. There was no way I could have predicted how her story would touch mine so directly.

We called these individual profiles "Triumph Over Tragedy." When I first introduced the series, I had to find a reason, or so I felt, to justify why a makeup artist was tackling more serious stories. After a while, the makeup aspect to it was dropped because what really resonated was giving voice to rare. We were inspiring a connection—an empathy. We were building an audience that cared.

That's precisely what we did, so I knew it could be done. And that's what I set out to do for NMO—on a global scale and with a life-and-death sense of urgency.

THE COLORS OF HOPE

As an entrepreneur and a visual thinker, coming up with a logo at the start of our marketing efforts was clearly in my wheelhouse. Still, I can remember first sitting down to design it, being hard-pressed to settle on a concept that would become the centerpiece of a communications platform. Why was branding our cause so important? Why did it matter so much that we embodied rare in our messaging?

In the business world, those questions might not even have to be asked. But in the medical field—and even for many philanthropists—

such essential aspects of communicating your goals to the world have often been ignored. Only recently have top medical schools and health-care policy programs started to enlist business-savvy professors to add instruction about marketing strategies for causes and cures.

In our case—starting at the time when there was no reference point at all for *what this mystery disease even was* and *who we were*—we needed a coat of arms, a flag, an image of some kind. We needed a true north for NMO to identify our mission. Branding ourselves as offering a rare approach to a rare disease gave us a powerful slogan. A strong step in the right direction. But because the real test of branding is how it instantly links a message to the mind, we needed an iconic logo to tell our story in the blink of an eye—without words.

A memorable brand identity could serve as a springboard to all media—from TV and commercial press to academic publications, to the creation of everything from our own films, books, and live lectures to streamed webinars and other digital content delivered with the latest technology. My intention was to weave a consistent message into every aspect of how we presented the Foundation and our vision to the world—starting with this emblem and its colors. Only, what would that be?

All I could think about as I sat staring at a blank page was my desire that the logo and the color palette convey a sense of hope and courage. I wanted the imagery to be uplifting and appear to be full of light. We were in the throes of feeling acute darkness, and I didn't want people to look at any of our materials and feel they were in the dark at all. That was me thinking like a makeup artist: light versus dark, highlight versus shadow, subtlety versus heaviness. What other concepts came to mind?

Community. Family. Love. Curing. Living. Growing. Organic. Life.

A story began to take form in images. There was shape, color, texture, pattern, and meaning. The logo was born.

Did it matter if anyone outside our circle knew of the symbolism of the tree branch with two leaves representing Bill and me, along with three other leaves representing Ali and her two brothers? Not to me. What mattered was that when anyone looked at the logo, our website, and our other multimedia materials that were framed in foliage of many shades of green, they saw the growth and healing that comes from being part of a natural and growing purpose. I wanted them to feel the light that would nurture new and miraculous ways to save and improve lives.

This kind of thinking was behind the logo and all the images, symbols, and icons that are part of the Guthy-Jackson Charitable Foundation (GJCF) brand. In many of our materials early on, I began including an image of a pair of hands cradling a small but sturdy bonsai tree with its roots reaching down into a handful of soil. At our events—such as Patient Days and Roundtables—our table centerpieces are potted bonsai trees, the most natural and green of them. Representing peace, balance, and harmony, masterpiece bonsai trees are rare and resilient. Bonsais are also known to stand for all that is good and correct in the world.

These basic symbols and subtle aspects of messaging also express healing properties. In hospital and clinic settings, more and more thought has been given to the impact of the art on the walls, the levels of lighting, the soft texture of blankets and therapeutic touch, the meditative sounds of nature and music in the background. They are comforting reminders that when focus is on wellness rather than illness, patients have better outcomes. They matter because medicine must treat the person, not the disease.

My belief is that how we speak to *all* our senses can dictate the difference between hope and futility, fear and courage, and between decline and true healing. When you set hope, courage, and light against darkness in such a way that positively engages all the senses, audiences will pay attention. Then it's up to you to tell your story and inspire those audiences to action.

MOVIE-MAKING FOR A CURE MOVEMENT

In a multifaceted, multipronged approach to marketing, one of the questions that kept me up at night in our early days (and into later years too) had no simple answer: how to connect head and heart in our storytelling about NMO. There were diverse audiences we needed to reach—from patients and their families to scientists and clinicians, from healthcare providers to policy makers and government agency regulators, from fellow philanthropists to industry leaders in the pharmaceutical and biotech sectors, and to potentially every member of the general public everywhere. If we were out to cause a revolutionary shift in consciousness toward curing diseases—rare and beyond—we had to tell the NMO story in the most universal terms possible. We had to share real and practical aspects of our approach as a model for evolving medicine and building a global cure movement that would unite these different audiences.

To begin to imagine how to do all that, I had to drill down into other questions. How could we find the right language to describe the complex science of NMO for those who weren't in the scientific world—and in a digital universe where attention spans were shorter than ever? How could we strike the right emotional tone, complete with narrative, for experts and potential allies to understand the urgency of finding a cure that had the potential to help cure so many other diseases? How could we do all that in dynamic, leading-edge media formats?

One of my first ideas was to create a YouTube video by putting together interviews with our leading NMO investigators. After all, one of the most frequent questions TV producers asked was if there was any B roll available for use on a segment. Classic catch-22. If I couldn't book a TV interview, how did we get them to generate that footage? So why not go the entrepreneurial route and, on our own, produce B roll that could be used for those TV bookings and our own purposes?

At the same time, I hadn't forgotten everything I'd learned from pioneering a different kind of look and feel in the infomercial industry. Back in 1991, at the first trade show ever hosted for the field (where I was first introduced to a certain Bill Guthy), I was honored to be named Best Female in an Infomercial. I used my acceptance speech to say that as marketers we had a responsibility to truth, and we needed to elevate our work by spending the money on higher-quality production values.

"Much of the public," I said back then, "associates what we do with snake oil salesmen, and that's *not* who we are."

Once a crusader, always a crusader.

"We're no less than any other top marketers," I insisted. "What makes us different is that we have this amazing challenge and opportunity to tell our true story in just twenty-eight minutes." If we were sharing celebrity testimonials and hearing from satisfied consumers achieving real results, we had to do more than just chalk up the numbers. "And what comes along with that is the responsibility to conduct ourselves with integrity and to deliver quality products that make a difference in people's lives, and provide customer service after sales have been made."

In other words, the "pitch" had to be personal, honest, *and* appealing—and was only the first step to success. Ditto with storytelling around NMO.

Of course, I wasn't looking to build an infomercial for solving a rare disease. But what I did want was to create the intimacy and intrigue that the best infomercials offer—only in a fraction of the time. And that's what I was sleeplessly mulling over . . . how to shoot a short film to combine the five elements of connection:

1. THE UNIVERSAL. That rare diseases affect everyone whether they know it or not

2. THE INFO. Why NMO is "the little disease that could" and how the science we were advancing could ultimately help save countless lives

3. THE PERSONAL. The story of living with NMO as told by patients, families, and caregivers, as well as researchers, doctors, and other stakeholders

4. THE PROFOUND. The real message of hope that connected to all the senses and would galvanize a cure

5. THE CALL TO ACTION. How each of us can play an active role in finding cures

I needed a collaborator. Easier said than done. But in these kinds of ventures, I knew to turn to those who really cared about me.

Thanks to friends of trusted friends, I found just the right person—
Jesse Dylan. Along with his team at Wondros Global, he was already
working on subject matter in the medical space. His mission was to create
content addressing issues of impact to everyone on earth.

Jesse—the son of Bob Dylan (yes, *that* Bob Dylan)—had produced
and filmed the iconic "Yes We Can" music video for Barack Obama's first
White House run. That historic mini-movie had gone viral in a nano-
second. Jesse understood the power of multisensory communications
that linked healing and activism. He was also tuned in to how studying
the bigger patterns in disease could help reveal bigger solutions. He recognized that decoding the molecular mechanisms in a rare disease like
NMO would translate into solving other diseases in global populations.

Jesse acknowledged, "Really complex ideas are hard to explain." What
he liked to do in his approach to filmmaking was to help organizations
hone their missions and translate them into something "bold and striking
like a commercial." The twist was incorporating the elements that really
explained the fundamental values of the cause.

From the moment I described our blueprint, Jesse's eyes lit up. This
was a big story with a big purpose. It had to be told, he agreed, and urgently. It was needed as an innovative model for accelerating solutions to
NMO *and* other diseases. He understood that our paradigm was different,
and could be captured in just a few phrases that could pass like a baton
from voice to voice: 1) get everyone in the room; 2) be sure they came from
diverse perspectives; and 3) make them share findings in real time. He insisted that ours was a model that could be easily referenced and replicated.

When Jesse mentioned that he had been contemplating a way to develop a search engine devoted to lesser-known information in the medical space—something like a "Google Med"—I responded that we would
soon be launching our own version of that kind of tool for downloading
digital education modules on our website. It would come to be known as
NMOPedia.

Toward the end of our meeting, Jesse pulled out a glossy poster and
unfolded it. The poster was covered in circles of all different colors and

sizes. Some looked like moons, others like suns, still others like stars. They all had smaller satellites orbiting around them. He called it a "disease-nome map"—a kind of atlas that showed how many human diseases exist in relation to one another. And right there on the atlas was a tiny, rare star—NMO—not far from MS and lupus. The atlas had not been created by doctors but rather by a thought leader outside the medical field.

The map was made in association with a paper titled "The Human Disease Network," and as fate would have it, the work had just been published in the *National Academy of Sciences* by researchers from the University of Notre Dame. One "Mother" helping another?

The beauty was the universal quest to understand disease connections and find cures. This was further confirmation that our movement would grow out of an understanding revealed by those connections between rare and common conditions. One cure would lead to another.

The images challenged my imagination. How could we tell the story of this tiny star (or maybe not so tiny) that had a superspecial quality that could allow it to emit much more light than just any star? How could we explain that NMO offered a rare opportunity for solutions, as a superstar? Could we visually map the story of how our research was connecting a solution for NMO to solutions for other diseases in which there is an immune identity crisis—from autoimmune disease to cancer, transplantation, wound healing, aging, and beyond?

Where would we begin?

TELLING IT LIKE IT IS

We decided to collaborate on a short four-minute film, *Pioneering a New Scientific Research Model*. Jesse and his team, a few of our own stars, and I brainstormed about who the storytellers should be and what we hoped they would say.

We quickly concluded that all we had to do was capture the truth about our collaborative approach so far to cure NMO, unfiltered and unscripted. Our diverse list of interviewees included a few patients and their family members—along with several of our best and brightest advisors: scientists and clinicians from the Mayo Clinic, University of Texas Southwestern, Stanford, Johns Hopkins, Harvard, and UCLA.

The mix of perspectives brought everything together—the right blend of head and heart, the highest hopes of medicine and human aspiration, the challenges of solving a complex rare disease, and a balance of reality and vision.

Not only did each of our medical experts explain in clear and basic terms where the science was taking us, but the optimism from everyone jumped off the screen. Dr. David Rosenman of the Mayo Clinic summed it up by saying that our work was transforming the understanding of NMO from a place where the field had been lit by a couple of flashlights to "the sun coming up." It was a new dawn for NMO patients and beyond.

Nothing could have been more powerful to the many audiences we needed to reach than hearing from patients themselves. The patients and family members who graciously appeared in our early videos were able to acknowledge how being engaged with a community working toward a cure had led to direct improvements to their health and well-being. That is the power of hope mixed with urgency that leads to momentum. And they weren't shy about reminding everyone to move even faster.

No matter what the cause for change might be, I knew that when trying to get the word out, celebrities almost have magical properties for attention-getting. Heeding that lesson, for our first video I was most fortunate to be able to include major stars who happen to be a couple of my dearest friends. One of them, Reese Witherspoon, had been on the journey with us from the very first night of Ali's eyeball headache. The second, Dustin Hoffman—along with his wife, Lisa—had implored me daily to ask for his help in any way, especially for helping to raise NMO awareness. The contributions from Reese and Dustin were so meaningful and heartfelt that we ended up developing a second short film, titled *Creating a New Dialogue About NMO*.

Once I saw the reach and impact of our first two films, I went on to produce several short movies with Jesse and his team. Some focused on heart. *Living with NMO*, for one, described patients' lives and challenges and hopes. This was one of the most emotional of the videos. Other films, like *Where Will the Cure Come From?*, went more deeply into the science of NMO breakthroughs and how everyone can be part of the cure. It empowered patients by helping them see how they held the cure within themselves—and urged them to consider participating in our CIRCLES research program.

Ali would be central to our later films as they began to focus on patients. With her own savvy storytelling instincts, Ali would also help me turn filmmaking challenges into opportunities. After one shoot that did not produce the footage I had hoped for, she suggested bringing in other imagery—while keeping the voiceover narration that I did like. Some crash-editing sessions later, and with the sweat and talent of some of our key advisors, we managed to create two films. *Ali Guthy & the Guthy-Jackson Charitable Foundation* was a live-action clarion call that featured her putting a public face on NMO. The other, *The NMO Story*, was an animated short film about my blueprint, and turned out to be one of the most effective videos we have for describing our work to date.

In 2012—a breakthrough year for all kinds of reasons—we achieved dramatic media momentum on many fronts. To take advantage of new opportunities and interest, I produced two additional films that could build on the momentum and help energize our growing presence in social media. One of them, *How Do We See in the Dark?*, was a celebration of the strengths of the NMO community. It was narrated by NMO patient Christine Ha, an attendee of our first Patient Day and a vocal patient advocate for NMO awareness. Christine had just won season three of Fox's *MasterChef*—the first blind cook to win that show, not to mention the only blind cook who had ever been a contestant on any cooking series. The metaphor of *How Do We See in the Dark?* was about how NMO patients were turning their own disadvantages into assets—just as Christine overcame blindness by using her senses of taste, smell, and touch to amaze everyone and win.

That was the story embodied by each of the countless NMO patients who made the choice to turn a limitation into a strength to achieve remarkable goals. This was the Power of Rare that I witnessed over and over within our NMO community.

The other film made that same year, *A Path to Progress*, was less a metaphor and more a global announcement that the NMO field was quickly evolving—and that we were writing its next chapters. All while making it relatable to everyone, the film covered major milestones achieved in the first four years of our work and previewed the radical developments ahead.

Even without naming the stages, they were all woven through the story of the film. Everyone on the journey could feel how fast we were moving. That picture was coming into bold reality as each blueprint phase unfolded or was about to unfold:

PHASE I. A New Scientific Tool Kit—Innovating the research nuts and bolts needed to enable breakthroughs for patients

PHASE II. Connect the Docs—Bringing the best and the brightest to the global NMO cure table

PHASE III. Industry & Agencies—Including industry, regulatory, and all stakeholders in the cure movement

And all this energy and momentum—this most intense, collaborative research to discover the new therapeutic targets—was moving us to the next place, Phase IV: Clinical Solutions. Our intensified focus would now be translating test tube discoveries into life-changing treatments with the development and delivery of improved medicines, therapeutic strategies, and diagnostic tools to ultimately cure NMO.

This was our continuous, relentless process that could be heard and felt in the voices of that film.

Dr. Amit Bar-Or, now of the University of Pennsylvania—a world-class expert on new therapeutics for NMO and other autoimmune diseases—summed it up by saying we were no longer the little engine that "could, would, and will" but the little engine that "*is.*" Several of our

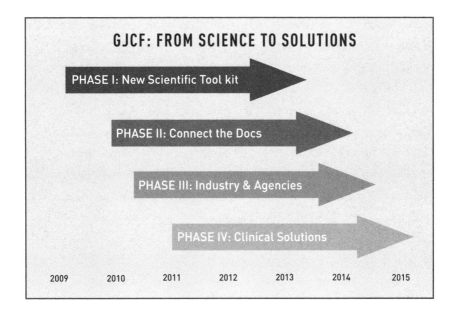

researchers and clinicians named the diseases that their work toward solving NMO was going to help—Parkinson's, Lou Gehrig's Disease (ALS), and other specific conditions that on their surface seem to have nothing to do with NMO.

Ali took us back to our roots and then described what progress meant to her: "My mom planted the seed for this foundation, and now it's grown into this beautiful, flourishing tree."

As I closed the film, my words put the emphasis squarely on the deliverables of all we were discovering and developing—"for the world."

It was a moment to exhale. Our work was really making things happen. Now, through the medium of movies, we were reaching new eyes and ears.

But I still wanted to go further—no surprise.

NMO TV

Whenever I think back to that producer who wanted to know "What else you got?" I have to silently thank her and the other media gatekeepers whose rejections motivated me to come up with new ways to get the NMO story out there—and told on our own terms. In the process, as a lot of different gates began to open, we multiplied our audience reach many times over.

Four years down the road, a new challenge arose that I believed could also be an opportunity—what could we do with all our amazing content?

In addition to our shorter, well-produced films, we had hundreds, if not thousands, of hours of video footage of interviews with experts. We had tapes of every Roundtable symposium, every summit meeting, every regional and international conference, every Patient Day, every breakout session, every Q&A panel, and every keynote address. And we had truly inspiring, unforgettable video logs made by patients telling their stories.

The more I thought about the value this library of information and inspiration held, the more I was sure there had to be some way to repurpose some of it. How? I began to resolve the answer with a series of other questions.

First, how hard would it be to expand one of our website's most trafficked tabs—"FAQs on NMO"—and include an individual video response from a leading authority on the particular subject being addressed? Not so hard. We already had them on film.

And second, why shouldn't we make all the content amassed available to everyone on the Internet? No reason whatsoever. Just as an example, take a Patient Day breakout session that was offered by Doctors Michael Yeaman, Scott Zamvil, and Larry Steinman on Simplifying the Science of NMO. In fifteen minutes, the three described and demonstrated in everyday language and relatable storytelling what was happening in the immune system of NMO. Anyone watching them live or on video would understand many of the following complex concepts, reduced to user-friendly images and terms:

• The communication of dendritic cells that function as the "scouts"—looking out for foreign antigens such as microbes or cancer cells that don't belong—and report back to the T cells through a cell-to-cell "molecular handshake."

- The key roles played by certain types of T cells that serve as the "conductors" of the immune system to make decisions about whether or not to attack an antigen.
- The work of B cells that make autoantibodies (proteins also called immunoglobulins), when antigens misidentified as foreign are detected—but can only do so if approved by T cells that also make the same mistake.
- The autoimmune disease spark that begins with binding of the autoantibody NMO IgG to the normal water channel AQP4 on the surface of astrocytes—cells in the central nervous system that support the health and wellness of neurons—and which appear to be targeted in NMO.
- The chain reaction fire of inflammation and demyelination that ensues when complement proteins are activated by the autoantibodies and injure or destroy cells to which the autoantibody has bound—and which in turn call in neutrophils and other white blood cells that rush to the site, amplifying inflammation and tissue destruction.
- How mistaken identity of normal antigen molecules like AQP4 causes immune cells to cross the blood-brain barrier (the junction that regulates what cells or molecules are allowed into or out of the central nervous system)—which leads to the loss of immune system regulation and then to disease.
- And how all these moving parts are being studied as biomarkers to diagnose NMO and prevent future relapses—and as targets for new drugs and ways to treat NMO—and as the hope of tolerization to ultimately cure it.

Yep . . . in our own Patient Day breakout session, somehow we got three luminaries of immunology to be part of a real-life play in which patients volunteered to be the main characters. One a T cell, another a B cell, another a dendritic cell, another a neutrophil, and so on—so that patients themselves could not only understand NMO but tell others about it. As Dr. Yeaman put it, "Patients created their own NMO mini–flash mob."

Another realization inevitably hit me: this crash course in autoimmune science could be used both by laypeople and researchers in other disciplines. So why wouldn't we share it?

Then, another brainstorm. We had the makings of NMO TV—a repository of knowledge generated by the brightest medical minds in the world. We were sitting on a virtual gold mine of material needed to change the landscape of rare.

The Foundation team and I went immediately to work to bring NMO TV to life. Today, between our foundation event chronicles, short films made in collaboration with Wondros, and our collection of interviews with experts and patients—plus all the media appearances Ali and I have made—NMO TV is home to more than 200 informative and inspirational videos.

This body of work that speaks both to head and heart has contributed mightily to the creation of our global grapevine. We have used our content to energize advocacy, education, and awareness. Our films have connected us to new partners and new friends.

The biggest takeaway for me was that if we were out to cause a revolutionary shift in consciousness toward curing diseases—rare or not—we had to tell the NMO story in the most universal terms possible. We had to share real and practical aspects of our approach as a model for changing medicine and building a global cure movement composed of all these different audiences.

We had to do it—for others, of course, but for ourselves as well.

SAVING EACH OTHER

One of the most generous gifts of advice I was given shortly after Ali's diagnosis was to keep a journal of the experiences and emotions to come. A loving friend of mine said, "Even if you can only write a few sentences, write a few lines every day. Whatever you need to say, paper will listen and you never have to show it to anybody else but you. Unless you decide otherwise."

At the time, with every minute devoted to setting up the Foundation—and juggling all those needs of marketing, money, molecules, and miracles—

baring my soul in any written form felt like pretty much the last thing I wanted to add to the plate.

But rather than ignore such sincere advice, I decided to just give it a try. At a time when Ali still didn't want to know what it was she had, I found that keeping a journal gave me a safe, private space to pour out my feelings and fears without having them overwhelm me.

Writing also helped me find my voice when I started ramping up our efforts to put NMO on the global map. Turning over all stones, I became a storytelling machine. As a note in drafting your own blueprint—once you find one opening, be ready to move through it with everything you have. It's like getting water from a well. Once you've primed the pump, let it flow.

There was no one piece of the marketing effort that led to a turning point. The key was not being intimidated. What a whirlwind. When I wasn't blogging under my own byline as a Mom on a Mission for the *Huffington Post*, I was talking to Bill Gates about Ali's "eyeball headache" and about the need for a cure movement to change the status quo toward rare "orphan" diseases. And when I wasn't speaking on a panel moderated by Tina Brown about becoming Dr. Mom, I was leading a TV camera crew from AARP's *My Generation* behind the scenes at one of our medical summits. At every opportunity I could find, I would talk or publish or be interviewed about NMO patients and game-changing researchers and industry leaders who were proving how our road to turning molecules into miracles was impacting all of medicine.

And when asked for evidence of that fact, I would simply point to the PubMed scoreboard. The published papers of our research grantees were beginning to multiply exponentially—and to be consistently featured in the top peer-reviewed medical journals. We knew we were getting traction when the numbers of citations in the published works of other renowned researchers started to skyrocket. The Foundation's sponsored research had risen to the top of PubMed's most cited science that was being applied and valued by investigators in publications of other diseases—at an uptick rate each year of 500 percent. That's not just a statistic to brag about; these publications would soon help set the stage for the first NMO clinical trials ever to be conducted.

PUBLISHED ITEMS IN EACH YEAR

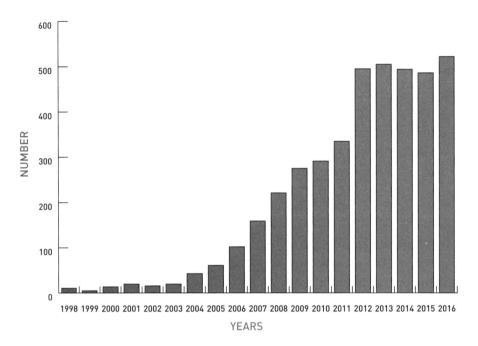

CITATIONS IN EACH YEAR

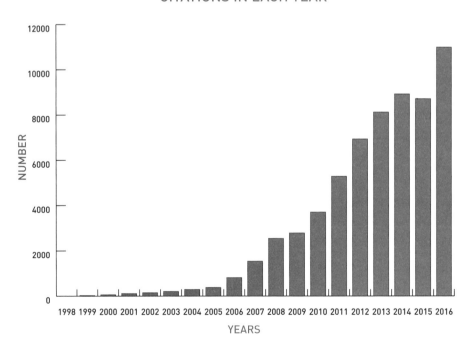

This was exciting. The more the word got out there, the better the chance for getting life-changing treatments to patients. And that was what we were all about.

We knew we had to be doing something right when, all of a sudden, we were asked for the first time to present findings at numerous international conferences on solving autoimmune diseases. Academic institutions and scientific organizations were soon including NMO in the name of their Demyelinating Disease department headings. This was more proof of a movement under way—making NMO highly recognizable among the leading medical authorities worldwide. Connecting through scientific publishing was even changing the estimate of how many NMO patients there were around the world—from a few thousand to potentially hundreds of thousands. In this light, as we would be learning more and more, rare was not so rare.

The challenge, still, was making inroads into everyday households. Even when we had broken through on a few media outlets, I knew we would need a way to sustain the momentum. Then a solution tapped me on the shoulder. A book. This most traditional form of calling cards would allow us to connect our personal NMO story to the personal lives of readers and audiobook listeners. Not to mention the media coverage that books garner.

Why was a book so important? For anyone crafting a blueprint for change, books are often a kind of manifesto. That's what I wanted—a platform for caring about rare. Besides, there's something about the written page that intimately connects readers to authors. I'd learned that from the two earlier books I'd written—one offering practical beauty advice (*Redefining Beauty*), and the other on empowerment and self-esteem (*Makeup Your Life*). For years afterward, I continued to hear from readers about how my stories of finding beauty in myself and others had made a difference in the way they saw themselves and the world.

Needless to say, a book about the universe assigning me a mission as a mom to unravel a mystery disease could offer that connection—and help shed more light on NMO. The obvious answer could come from the journal I'd been keeping. Or my "Momoir," as I liked to think of it.

With the plan to go ahead and tell Ali about what I'd written, I decided to call the book *Saving My Daughter, Finding Myself* and hoped she would approve.

Nothing could have prepared me for her response when I mentioned I had been writing all along to keep track of the journey. As I recall, it was a crisp autumn day, and Ali—then seventeen years old, already a senior in high school and captain of the tennis team that she was about to lead to a magical championship—had just come home from practice. On hotter days and during matches, Ali had to maintain a strict regimen that involved discreetly being iced down during breaks so as not to become overheated—which was thought to contribute to NMO attacks or worsening symptoms. So after I asked how practice had gone and Ali reassured me that all was well, I broached the subject of my Momoir.

Ali only beamed and then said she would be right back, returning moments later from her room holding a diary of her *own*! Unbeknownst to me, she had been keeping her own reflections over the tumultuous years following her diagnosis. She showed me her first entry, in which she described her diagnosis as an autoimmune condition that would affect how she lived her life, but—"Don't worry about the disease thing, it's not like I have cancer or anything, it's just a little bump in the road for me."

Her first entry also included this P.S.: "Always remember to love Mom, she cares so much and does so much for you, she is really someone special."

There was no stopping the tears as she showed me other excerpts that brought up my own memories that were sometimes in distinct contrast to her recollections.

Over the course of a few pages, I witnessed Ali's heart there on paper—funny, loving, and visionary—all coming to life as she evolved from girlhood into a young woman. Though she described taking a more active role as a patient advocate, I did notice how she would safeguard herself from talking about her feelings—and instead spend more time making observations about the blueprint we were creating with the Foundation:

I have to say that my mom is not just out to change how research is done but also to challenge the terrible unfairness that exists when it comes to access to great medical care. She has made a reformer out of me. . . . It's just that I feel so strongly that access to medical treatment shouldn't be so heavily reliant on financial status. And part of what Mom is doing with the Foundation is coming at that problem. She is only one person. She can't change the entire world on her own. But in my view, she may just prove that the medical field can be a more accessible place for everyone.

All this time, I had been careful never to project my fears onto Ali or let her even suspect that every milestone she reached was a defiance of the prognosis we had once been given. But her journal revealed how well she knew me: Ali knew my fears and wasn't going to take them on for herself. Instead, she was going to make every moment of life count—for herself and her fellow NMO patients.

That's when I had a revelation—that as much as my motive was to save her by curing NMO, she was saving me from giving in to the debilitating force of fear. Through the incredible power of love for each other—revealed and reinforced through this rare journey traveled side by side—we were overcoming the odds together.

Ali had come a long way from the "ignorance is bliss" wish to her role as an advocate spreading the gospel of "knowledge is power." Not to mention the fact that her writing was poignant, original, and just beautiful.

So when Ali suggested that we give both journals to an editor to look into the possibility of weaving our voices together, I couldn't have been more thrilled.

The result was a rare coauthorship of the book we decided to call *Saving Each Other: A Mystery Illness—A Search for a Cure—A Mother Daughter Love Story*. It was one of, if not the most, emotionally fulfilling collaborations I could have ever been given the gift of receiving.

The book was completed against the extraordinary backdrop of major milestones in Ali's life as she moved from surviving to thriving, from defying all the worst predictions to graduating high school with rare honors and heading off to four years of college for even more.

None to my surprise, in October 2012, publicity for the book kicked off the media momentum that brought NMO in from the wings and onto center stage. We were featured separately and together in area newspapers, magazines, and on outlets like the *Huffington Post*, *Teen Vogue*, and on *The Ellen DeGeneres Show*, as well as on a crazy radio junket that broadcast into the homes of many remote and rural listeners who were among the households toughest to reach.

In every appearance or interview we did in connection to the book, my goal was to communicate a delicate balance of urgency and hope. Ali, at my side or on her own, picked up on those cues and added her own blend of reality and positive possibility. One of the most telling responses came during an interview when she was asked how NMO affected her every day.

Ali's answer must have resonated for many patients not just with NMO but with other rare autoimmune or other diseases thought to be "incurable." She explained:

I may look like a normal college student walking around campus, but that doesn't change the fact that I wake up every morning knowing I have NMO. I wake up, and go to class, and have breakfast, and hang out with friends, but that doesn't change the fact that at any moment, I could be brought to my knees by the crippling pain of an attack and be rushed to the nearest hospital. When people look at me, they don't see that side. Just because I'm not blind (although I almost was) and not in a wheelchair does not mean I'm not directly affected by this disease. I still lie awake in fear that all of a sudden my back will start to hurt or my legs will go numb as they have several times before. But the important thing to remember is that there is always a silver lining. Today, I am okay, and I will keep moving forward and living my life just as I've always planned to, and nothing will stop me from doing just that.

And then came the moment when the two of us strode in together to sit down and talk about *Saving Each Other* on *The Ellen DeGeneres Show*—which at the time was reaching as many as 4.5 million viewers a show. And that's daytime. Ellen DeGeneres, a friend I can count as one of my very dearest, had not only been on this journey from the start with us, and knew where we had begun and where we were headed—and how our approach was different—but she had read the book and was able to rouse viewers to care and to act.

One of the most emotional moments of the interview came toward the beginning when Ellen reminded me of the passage in which we were told that Ali might not live to see her eighteenth birthday, and now here she was, almost nineteen, and going strong.

And Ali promptly added, "And I'm not going anywhere."

Then the focus shifted to me, and it was my turn to talk about the Power of Rare—about the strides we were making for all NMO patients, the challenges of misdiagnosis, and how our work could provide the keys to the kingdom for the next generation of treatments and cures for NMO, autoimmune diseases, and a host of more common illnesses.

Thanks to one classic marketing lesson I'd learned from my media past, I knew that when you only have a short time to get your message out, it's good to have those bullets ready to fly off the tip of your tongue. And Ellen, who is one of the most quick-witted and caring people on the planet, was ready to make sure I got those talking points out there for everyone to hear.

That experience again reminded me that I was grateful for the rejections received early on. Without them I wouldn't have been ready for the opportunities that came later. The old adage that all publicity is good publicity is just not true. You have only a few shots to get it right when you land your mystical fifteen minutes of fame—so make them count.

When you have a message that connects, you can extend those fifteen minutes indefinitely.

At last, we had a spotlight, we were telling our story, and we had a lot more to say. For everyone in our NMO community, having a book in hand meant we were no longer behind the curtain.

In the coming months and weeks, our foundation team tracked a marked uptick in our website's Internet traffic and in new contacts from around the world. Experts began to recalculate the numbers of NMO patients worldwide yet again.

This was a reminder too of how many more patients were counting on us to change the course of the NMO future. That was sobering. And so too were the number of patients who were sight-impaired—one of the more unfortunate and cruel tolls our NMO family members had to suffer. With that in mind, and wanting to include everyone, I was able to convince the publisher to quickly produce an audiobook—which was lovingly received in our own patient community.

We reached out to all and just kept rolling—doing interviews that ranged from women's health issues to philanthropy to mother-daughter relationships to the power of patient advocacy and the need to care for the caregivers. Turning over all stones.

Soon enough we began to receive requests from authors of new books in the works about rare diseases and novel cures. One of them in which Ali and I participated for a chapter on NMO was *The Healing Cell* by Robin L. Smith, MD; Msgr. Tomasz Trafny; and Max Gomez, PhD. This book reflected a huge step forward regarding the openness of spirituality to meet science—and included a special message from Pope Benedict XVI. In a stunning turn of events, my miraculous daughter and I would soon be invited to speak at a Vatican conference.

For a mother like me, who had each of my three babies blessed in many religions, the invitation to be in the circle of the Pope was a gift in itself. With all my prayers, I had to think this was a step closer to being heard, as the saying goes—"From my lips to God's ears."

But even God sometimes has other plans, as I would have to soon face.

I am inspired daily by my work with individuals with NMOSD. The power of their stories, their resilience and their struggles has a strong impact on everyone involved in their care. The power of these rare individuals is to promote increased awareness that leads to early diagnosis, effective treatment and eventually a cure for NMOSD.

—Nancy L. Sicotte, MD, FAAN

Professor and Vice Chair for Education,
Director Neurology Residency Training Program
Director Multiple Sclerosis Program,
Department of Neurology,
Cedars-Sinai Medical Center, Los Angeles

TURNING EMPATHY INTO ENTERPRISE

As I continued to push the boundaries we had to cross in our cure move-ment, I would continue to raise the stakes on the familiar *M*s needed to keep the Foundation firing on all cylinders. And more. If I had learned anything, as Dr. Yeaman was quick to remind me, the recurring theme was finding a way to make NMO personal to everyone.

True. Whether you are fund-raising or seeking activism or connect-ing to advocates or industry partners or the general public, I agreed with his point that to engage lasting commitment to a cause, it has to matter to them—and in a firsthand way.

How did we go about building that rare, powerful connection of em-pathy?

Dr. Yeaman has a way with words that speak to many audiences and turn rare concepts into realistic and relatable callings. He explained there is a world of difference between sympathy and empathy. Sympathy is like watching someone suffer from the sideline while offering well-intentioned but hollow good wishes. Empathy is more about getting in the game—knowing from experience how it feels to walk a mile in that person's shoes.

Here were his suggestions for revealing empathy: 1) there had to be a relatable story that illuminated empathy not sympathy; 2) there could only be such a story of empathy if those who would join the cause felt it affected them too—personally—directly or indirectly; 3) advocates and partners would only feel directly affected if there was a real health con-nection linking them and those with the diagnosis—even for NMO, em-pathy could connect those who were at risk for such a condition, as well as relatives and loved ones; or 4) that biological link could be sharing a com-mon thread that might be, as one example, other autoimmune diseases or a more common issue caused by immune dysfunction—such as cancer or infection—which at one point or another will affect nearly everyone.

Science meets soul. The circle of empathy surrounding NMO was growing larger and larger. And that was something I could believe in.

I knew the power of empathy would be significant when it came to our outreach for new and bigger funding streams. That hadn't mattered to us before. For the first phase of our work, our blueprint had gone against that tradition. Why?

Just glance over one calendar page of the Beverly Hills registry for fund-raisers, galas, charity auctions, entertainment benefits, and all manner of celebrity-studded social functions for a multitude of worthy causes that happen almost daily. Bill and I didn't want to use that model. First of all, we didn't want to tap our friends' wallets when they were supporting many of those worthy causes. Rather, we had chosen to fund the early phases of our mission ourselves. There wasn't a day that I didn't thank our good fortune in business that allowed Bill to write the big checks that made our work possible.

Now that we were entering Phase IV—Clinical Solutions—we were ready to do outreach to collaborate with new partners, donors, and allies. To that end, we had established a sister organization (The Guthy-Jackson Research Foundation, Inc.) that made it possible for more corporations and organizations to donate to our mission. Regardless of the sources of the contributions—from public and private organizations or from individuals who are family members, friends, colleagues, or concerned citizens—we would maintain a strict policy that 100 percent of all monies received were put directly toward NMO research.

It was easy for me to see that marketing and fund-raising would rely on finding empathy—not sympathy. How did that connect molecules to miracles? Well, that was where the rubber was going to meet the road: we would need to convey how the many efforts in just a few short years had produced science that was now ready to be turned into medicine. To date, none of the treatments in use for NMO had received regulatory approval in any country. That fact brought with it far too much guesswork for clinicians, trial and error for patients, and awful insurance red tape for all.

Yet we were now at a place to change that. It was a new day.

And turning points bring great clarity. The time had come to transform laboratory molecules into miracle cures by defying all the traditional barriers standing in the way of industry-sponsored drug trials.

When I began my outreach to industry and regulatory partners, I was told by many—and in no uncertain terms—that this would be very slow going and could not happen with the same collaborative approach we'd developed in the research space.

After hearing all the practical and undeniable reasons why that may have been the case up to that point, I shrugged them off. Maybe that was naive. Or maybe that was the mother lion in me insisting it could and would be done. We had the molecules—the science of NMO—ready to roll. And we had the miracles—Ali and all the resilient and unstoppable NMO patients. We had a growing movement committed to the cures. We had a story of possibility that was going to matter to millions.

Looking back at everything that went into the blueprint having to do with the four *M*s, I realize just how much I learned—and am still learning—about how to tell the story of rare in a way that speaks all languages. Even in a fast-paced and moving-target media landscape, there are some timeless and universal lessons worth remembering and sharing:

- When challenged by rejection from those who don't buy your pitch, revise, reinvent, retool—or move on to someone else who gets it. Use the energy of disinterest as fuel for making your message count the next time.

- Even great causes need great marketing. And great marketing is all about storytelling—fresh, clear, honest, and passionate. In telling your story, connect others to why your urgent issue matters to them—find that common ground.

- The wisdom of the immune system—know thyself—illustrates a best-kept secret for what makes the best stories unforgettable: rare truths can reach big audiences if made relatable.

- You don't need an MBA to understand how messaging matters in any market. Your "molecules" are the essence of your truths—and your "miracles" are the good they can do. Brand

your mission with these marks, and your audience will remember long after.

- Help media to get your story out there. Provide tools and assets. Make it simple—and be prepared once a story gains
traction to follow up with the next chapter.

- Marketing is a means not an end—be ready to walk the walk.
Getting the word out and connecting rare can build a movement. But you need to turn energy into action to change lives.
In the end, you need people to do more than care. You need
movement.

We had tossed the pebble of our story into the global waters, and the
ripples were radiating. I felt, in return, that the message of saving each
other had begun to reach everyone.

Now our cure movement needed to find those other partners to agree
and apply their skills alongside ours. That vision was in the blueprint all
along.

Alone we can do so little—

together we can do so much.

—*Helen Keller*

CHAPTER 6
_____

BRAVE NEW PARTNERSHIPS

Back in the beginning of creating our NMO journey, I had a vision of forming an advisory board made up of outsiders from different sectors of industry and government agencies. If we were to solve a complex disease that involved many moving parts—from the immune system to academic research to industry investment to regulatory approval—this concept was really just a natural extension of getting everyone in the room. The idea made great sense . . . *in theory*. However, as I had to learn, there were all kinds of reasons why forging these unconventional relationships would not be quick or simple, and would require creative new thinking.

From our focus and our need to be real, we had to pay attention to the changing face of the business of medicine. We had to acknowledge the harsh realities and figure out how to navigate them anyway—one of the most important themes that threads through my blueprint. On one hand, the business of medicine, more and more, was becoming the driver for turning test tube findings into life-saving treatments. On the other hand, venturing into any aspect of drug development meant dealing with the turbulent winds affecting invention and intellectual property—which often provide the very returns on investment that allow breakthrough medicine to occur at all.

In this climate, I also knew perceptions mattered. We had to pay attention to the fact that conventional biomedical research and commercial
drug development have had very different histories. In the past, the common perceptions were that academic research efforts were in the pursuit of the truth, whereas biotech and pharmaceutical companies were
in pursuit of the money. In reality, the lines between discovery and development had been blurred to the point that they probably no longer
existed. Academic teams were now venturing into drug development and
new start-ups were investing powerful technology and their own bank-
rolls into every biomedical niche. The name of the game was assembling
the best combination of players to bring life-saving treatments and cures
to the clinic.

We would need to bring every skill and every sector to the table, from
discoverers to drug developers to regulatory approvers. We had to do so
with transparency and honesty that would be clear to patients and their
loved ones. We would need to build bridges over valleys of death.

And first there were more tough questions to be answered. How do
you convince hard-nosed competitors to become allies? How do you inspire nontraditional partnerships to maintain competition and connect
them to the same team? How do you motivate them to move at an unprecedented pace that dogma says just cannot be done?

These questions have everything to do with the Power of Rare. They
go hand in hand with other questions I'd asked all along: How do you
motivate thinking and action to cure the incurable? How do you make
the impossible *possible*?

The answers reminded me to start thinking about the "who" even as
I worked on the "how."

Whatever the challenge, I have looked for the best people who have
that unique mind-set or skill set and who also recognize opportunity.
That wasn't going to change when I started to look for the right decision
makers in the private and public sectors to collaborate with each other
and us. My mission would be to convince each of these rare leaders of

an even rarer opportunity not to be missed—how the profit potential of developing therapies for NMO could lead to drugs for diseases with much bigger numbers. But the message and the meaning were about more than money. And as much as the impact would save countless lives, it went even beyond NMO into the realm of changing the world of medicine.

The key to revolutionizing these brave new partnerships would be in making the connections between our goals and theirs. But there were still huge steps to be taken first.

SURVIVING THE CRUCIBLE OF DEVELOPMENT

Before we could come up with an effective strategy for getting some of the big industry players to even have a conversation about rare, I had to be mindful of a tangled web of historic barriers to all new or improved drug development—especially for all the "orphans." I still cringe at the memory of learning the term "Valley of Death" as a reference to the twelve to fifteen years it can take for one drug to go from a research lab breakthrough to life-changing medicine for a patient.

Twelve to fifteen years? Are you kidding me?

Everyone calls it the Valley of Death because the perils of the process are that real. After billions of dollars spent every year, only 50 in 5,000 (or just 1 percent of the drugs that first go into preclinical testing) will end up moving into human testing. And to make matters worse, only one of those fifty drugs will ever be approved for patient use. You are reading that right—just 1 in 5,000 promising test tube discoveries make their way through the drug development process to regulatory approval. That's .02 percent. Not quite impossible odds—but nearly.

I would never accept those limitations—not when we had the science to give Ali and all NMO patients better options that could change and restore their health and allow them to live full, healthy lives.

My battle lines were drawn.

How impossible was it to get past the nightmare of the Valley?

Early on, Dr. Yeaman had reminded us of the realities: "Even the greatest discovery or most promising cure in the laboratory will never save one life if it does not endure the crucible of development." Intellectual property and patenting. Non-dilutive and venture-stage funding. Preclinical optimization. Multiple phases of human clinical trials. And, of course, the long, slow walk toward regulatory approval. He added that in between each of these steps were challenging hurdles. So not just one Valley of Death where a discovery could die—but potential valleys between *each* hurdle.

And over each chasm was the narrowest of planks that would need to be crossed or countless patients' lives and hundreds of millions of dollars could be lost.

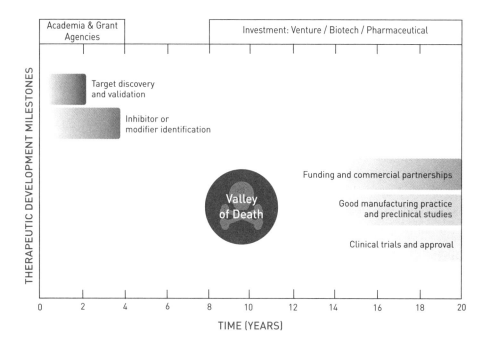

The challenge, to put it in old-school terms, was to learn to talk the talk and then walk the walk. And we could. Bill and I had the business savvy to know that the best deals were those in which each stakeholder stood to gain. In terms of medical development, we also had the advantage of advisors who had firsthand experience in founding companies that turned science into medicine.

It had been part of our vision and strategy all along to have those multifaceted leading medical lights who understood the business of medicine. That was in the blueprint—knowing we would do far more than observe and cheer from the sideline. We saw the need to be in the trenches not just with researchers and clinicians but now in pushing forward with industry professionals and agency officials. Those were the brave new partnerships that would change and save lives.

To help create these new alliances, our advisors conceived of a novel road map for solving NMO that quickly turned heads. They published a first-of-its-kind manuscript titled "Integrative Continuum: Accelerating Therapeutic Advances in Rare Autoimmune Diseases." The paper appeared in one of the most cited of all medical journals, namely the *Annual Review of Pharmacology and Toxicology*. It was the first paper to provide a hyperlink to a real-time, interactive immunology tool kit called "Visualizing NMO." This feature allowed every reader to become a sort of user immersed interactively in the structure of the immune system. They could visualize the precise molecular and cellular pathways in NMO—and experience how these pathways and their components could be targets for drug repurposing or innovation to solve the disease. This paper laid out a practical, transformational plan for how each of the different stakeholders could and should work together to cure NMO.

One of the main points in this revolutionary paper was how solving NMO meant facing a *wider* Valley of Death than most diseases faced in terms of drug development. A simply rendered figure that the authors included said it all: there, between basic research funded by academic and grant agencies on the one hand and investment by venture, biotech, and pharmaceutical interests on the other hand loomed the dreaded Valley.

But the paper also told another story. By laying out specific ways to accelerate therapeutic advances, there was now real hope for getting to the other side of the Valley—alive. This was a big deal for all the sufferers waiting for desperately needed drug development—and especially for the rare and the orphaned.

That much I knew well from a glance at the history of those disease classifications.

EMBRACING THE ORPHANS

The image and feeling of the word "orphan" has always bothered me. Even though I was not literally an orphan, hearing it tended to bring up a feeling of abandonment and unfair neglect that somehow felt personal. Maybe it has something to do with spending the first three months of my life in a hospital—and not being able to bond with either of my parents at a time when my survival was touch-and-go. Or maybe it has to do with being a child of divorce and hearing my father say to me at age nine that he was giving my sister and me up for adoption. In my young brain that was something that only happened to orphans.

Flash-forward to the world of curing a rare disease.

When I learned the numbers that showed how little funding rare diseases got for drug development from government and industry, I disliked the term "orphan" even more. In this sense, when a disease is labeled with the orphan stigma, it often reflects a lack of interest, funding, and priority to support finding a cure.

There are important differences between a rare disease and an orphan disease. Rare diseases are defined objectively by the numbers. For example, in the United States, diseases that affect fewer than 200,000 people are considered rare diseases. Orphan diseases, on the other hand, are much more subjectively defined. An orphan disease may be rare or not, but it has been relatively ignored in terms of resources and effort to find solutions. The National Institutes of Health (NIH) and the Food and Drug Administration (FDA) mainly use the term "orphan" for a disease that has been neglected by science and medicine for a variety of reasons. It may come down to the numbers. Orphan diseases are often rare too. And rare diseases frequently don't receive the awareness, funding, or expertise that more common diseases do. It may come down to futility. Some orphan diseases are those for which no good therapy has been found, despite all best intentions.

I remember hearing the example of the cancer therapeutic drug ipilimumab, which received orphan drug status from the FDA in 2004 for its development. Was cancer classified as a rare disease? No. However, the drug had been developed for a type of cancer that had few to no treatment options, which convinced a panel of regulatory experts to afford it orphan drug status to incentivize and speed development of solutions.

Clearly, I could see that the challenges in research and development were mighty for rare and orphan diseases. Like being between a rock and a hard place. The causes of these diseases might be well-known in terms of a genetic or other factor gone wrong. But when too few individuals were afflicted, making the case for the investment of money and labor-intensive time could be difficult.

And yet here's the rub—when you begin to look at the numbers of people rare diseases affect, they start to feel anything but rare. Let's revisit some of the numbers mentioned earlier. Around the world, 350 million people suffer from a rare disease. In the US alone, nearly 30 million people—that's about 1 in 10—are living with a rare, debilitating, and often life-threatening illness. The National Organization for Rare Disorders (NORD) reports there are 7,000 rare diseases, most without cures, and 95 percent have precious few or no treatments. Half of those afflicted with those rare disorders are children and adolescents. All the more reason to feel anguish about orphan status.

Rare diseases are complex. Many take a massive toll on our healthcare system. On top of that is the toll they impose on patients and families: frequent misdiagnosis, limited access to specialized medical expertise, the reduction or loss of employment due to health issues, an inability to qualify for disability compensation, and costs that are often denied by insurance and that can soar to the hundreds of thousands of dollars per year. As if the disease was not hard enough, these burdens only add to the cruelties of the illnesses that affect lives unfairly.

For most of the last century, there were vanishingly few incentives for pharmaceutical companies to invest money or time to develop new drugs or even to run clinical trials to repurpose existing medications that *might* only help a limited number of patients. When you consider the billions in profits that can be made with drugs that achieve blockbuster status by treating millions of patients—say for a new cholesterol drug or an antidepressant—you see why drugs for orphan diseases can be low on the priority list. The bottom line for most drug companies is that it would be too difficult to recover the costs of research and development for small groups of patients who are often spread out geographically across the globe.

None of this is said to point blame at the pharmaceutical industry. These companies have shareholders, and the executives have fiduciary responsibilities. I get it. But drug company CEOs have families too—and some of those families have members afflicted by rare diseases. I had to believe there was a way to connect the minds and hearts of these leaders to patients and families suffering from NMO, and show them how solving NMO was bigger than just one rare disease.

Were there any other incentives? Some. They had been long in coming, however.

As I learned, the growing concern from the medical community had led to Congress passing the Orphan Drug Act in 1983. To encourage drug companies to make the investment, the act created tax credits, extended market exclusivity, offered research assistance, and simplified some of the steps for attaining regulatory approval. At least that was a start. *Except* that over the next thirty years, only 326 of 18,000 therapies studied as possible treatments for rare diseases went on to receive approval by the FDA. The good news was that many of the treatments that emerged were for diseases that literally had no drug options. But that still left some 17,000-plus attempts by the wayside—and millions of rare patients desperately waiting for help.

Something revolutionary had to happen. The culture had to change.

Spurred on by rare patients and their advocates, Congress again acted to promote research and development in the rare disease space. This time they passed the Rare Diseases Act of 2002. As a result, the NIH responded by creating the Rare Diseases Clinical Research Network to "address the unique challenges of research on rare diseases." Seven years later, nineteen different rare diseases had received NIH funding for clinical research.

Great. Things were finally moving forward. But there was still a huge problem—these measures addressed some of the symptoms but didn't get to a cure; they didn't change the drug development *system* when it came to rare diseases.

Our deep dive into NMO and rare disease drug development also revealed a bigger story: the challenges of turning science into medicine affected *everyone*. This was true at a time when the rapid advances in the laboratory were outpacing the development and regulatory systems to turn them into treatments and cures. As journalist David Bornstein wrote in a 2011 article for the *New York Times*: "An ocean of research is producing cures and treatments by the drop."

The remedy? According to Mr. Bornstein, the solution to surviving the Valley of Death for rare and common diseases alike would be to find a way to get the diverse players together to "focus on common goals and deliberately align their efforts" and then devise a "targeted and methodical approach."

Easy to say—hard to do.

A BRIDGE ACROSS THE VALLEY

All these constraints brought out the warrior in me. Sometimes I thought of myself as a fearful warrior, true, but that didn't keep me from rolling up my sleeves to build a new kind of bridge across the canyon of death and failure.

We had already taken a major step by making sure that every research grant funded was tranched—as in tied to milestones that had to be reached for funds to be released before moving on. Of course, this was how we kept laser-beam focus on moving science toward the clinic to help patients. Second, even though we were providing millions of dollars in funding, we continued to maintain our policy that all intellectual property would be retained by the inventors and their institutions. That was our research model: we catalyzed breakthroughs—no strings attached. This strategy, as we saw all along, rewarded those who made discoveries worth patenting to earn future resources to drive future breakthroughs. Third, and again, this was in our research blueprint, was to build collaboration in the precompetitive space. That is, consensus-building and cooperative research can be greatest among otherwise competing stakeholders *before* you get to commercial development. This approach harnessed the best intentions of each of the minds and hearts in the room—and leveraged healthy competition when the time was right for them.

Consider the real-world situation. As I had come to know all too well, there are many hurdles before a promising drug candidate can even begin the gauntlet of clinical trials. Once at that starting gate, Phase I trials begin—which are all about safety and are usually conducted with healthy volunteers. Phase II trials focus largely on safety in patients who have the target disease, and on how to dose the drug for a best chance of effectiveness. Then come what are called the pivotal Phase III clinical trials. These are the trials that most of us think of when we hear whether a drug works or not. Phase III trials test for effectiveness relative to safety, and the results of this phase of study are provided to the regulatory agencies for review and possible approval.

Oh, but that's not all.

The regulatory agencies consider safety to be the top priority in testing any new drug or device. Add to this the need for a new drug to prove its effectiveness, and the road is long and winding. Each phase could be more than a couple years, in addition to the years leading to and following a phase. Were we talking *twenty* years?

And then there is the dilemma of the patent cliff. When a discovery is made and patented, a clock starts that only gives the inventors so much protected time to move from test tube to treatment. This is the period during which investors provide resources in hopes of achieving an approved drug product. But let's say that time is eighteen years, and let's say a drug takes twelve years from patent to approval—and costs $250 million dollars to achieve this goal. That would mean there are only six years of patent life remaining—the time left for the investors to recover their costs. At year eighteen, that drug reaches what is called its patent cliff, where protection falls away, and with it the exclusive right to manufacture and sell the drug. So even the best candidate drugs must walk a tightrope over the Valley between time and money.

And to add an even greater challenge to the mix: all these risks are amplified when it comes to investing in drugs for rare "orphan" diseases.

The more I learned about the process, the more the Valleys kept multiplying. Orphan diseases, again, present special hurdles to drug development. For example, the rarer the disease, the fewer patients there are to enroll in clinical trials. From a risk versus reward standpoint, companies are often hesitant to invest large sums of funding into developing a treatment for a rare disease given the limited return on investment. Yes, saving lives pays moral dividends. No question. But revenues pay real bills.

One note of hope came from the fact that orphan diseases had earned certain special privileges in the drug-development process. Basically, when a company decides to pursue the process of clinical trials for a rare disease, it can seek "orphan status" for its drug candidate. Gaining this status means that if the drug is eventually approved, the company has greater protection from competition—for a defined period of time, that helps in the recovery of investment costs.

Putting all that information together, we understood the rules of the drug-development chess match—and our challenge was to leverage them to bring otherwise competing stakeholders together to find solutions for the rare and orphan disease NMO.

"Was there any hope . . . in time?" I had to ask.

Dr. Yeaman confirmed there was, as long as specific challenges were met: "Great scientific insight, entrepreneurial savvy, technological mastery, clinical acumen, and good luck—or . . ."

I held my breath. As we all know, belief in a favorable outcome can be powerful, but luck is not a strategy. Something much more tangible was required. Especially if it meant revolutionizing a system that countless others had already complained about and had tried to reinvent. "Or . . . ?" I asked.

"Or a once-in-a-generation convergence of science, technology, industry, regulatory agencies, and patient connectivity," he answered. And as he continued, it became clear that we were entering such a window of opportunity.

So much so, Dr. Yeaman predicted that the ripple effect of our research and blueprint would lead to unique partnerships between us and other entities not used to working together—and in turn would afford time and cost efficiencies to dramatically but responsibly speed progress.

Still, I wasn't sure how to open the right doors to make our case—but I was sure NMO and other orphan diseases needed us to succeed.

I held fast to my vision to create our own Industry Council that would work with us—and each other. *Except*—no surprise here—if we were going to revolutionize the process of translating medicine from "bench to bedside," more needed to be done to replace the orphan stigma with a truer appreciation of rare diseases. We had to shine a light on the secrets that a rare disease like NMO could reveal about how our bodies work that more common diseases could not.

THE GIFT OF RARE: EXCEPTION PROVES THE RULE

"Rare" often has a mystical and noble feel when it comes to the natural world. We read headlines of the sighting of some great ocean giant that stirs images of myths and legends. Or the uncommon plant that blooms just once a century. And then there is the infinitely rare bird.

Here is one paradox of rare. It's not that a thing is so rare that makes it magical. It's what rare teaches about all that's around us every day. That's the magic. The rarest of species reveal secrets for how to survive and adapt. They're mirrors into the mystery of what we have yet to learn about the more common.

As I've come to understand it, this concept can best be described as "the exception proves the rule."

Studying rare teaches many truths—including the fact that in the fight-or-flight realities of nature, there are no free passes. I know that from my own experience. Over time, each life learns to best cope with the conditions it faces. True. But when change happens, those best suited to adapt survive. Change is the great disrupter—it selects for rare resilience.

Rare is the exception that proves the rule.

Let me put this in a personal context. Sometimes I walk along the beach and spot changes brought about by the tides and the winds that shape the water and earth in ways that can only be known over time. The same secret knowledge can be learned by paying attention to the rare sea star that shows itself only in chilly morning tide pools. Or the rare fire crab that hides until the harvest moon lights the autumn sky.

You ask yourself how these creatures became so different from everything around them. You follow the clues—you feel the connections. Then it comes clear: you realize in an instant how *all life* tells its own story of adaptation.

The exception *is* the rule.

So why doesn't this same appreciation of "rare" extend to the world of human diseases? Not just by industry—but by everyone. Could it be as simple as bad marketing? Or was it because of an outdated way of measuring impact rather than looking at the value of rare diseases more closely? As Dr. Yeaman has pointed out, "A rare autoimmune disease is actually proof of how the immune system *should* work. Of course, solving NMO will help crack the code of other autoimmune diseases—but it will also open the door to curing cancer—and everything in between."

For those of us in the trenches, early on NMO taught the lesson of how much we could learn about all immune dysfunction through a disease with a small population of patients. We had turned the curse of rare into a power squared that was radically pushing the science forward in understanding much broader aspects of the immune system. The potential gave us this unique vantage point for developing therapies that could even reset the immune system from disease to health—not just in NMO but in all autoimmune and other diseases.

Still, valuing rare and spreading the gospel of why it mattered—part of my blueprint—was only the start to bringing in partners who didn't share the same value. Yet. Even so, a revolution was afoot. And thanks to a lot of legwork, we managed to change the trajectory of drug development in the treatment of NMO.

The moment that shifted the tide was an exception to the rule too.

The approach taken by GJCF in attempting to cure NMOSD should serve the entire orphan disease community. It captures the prototype of an exception making the rule and the unusual guiding us past the distracting trees.

—Terry J. Smith, MD
Frederick G.L. Huetwell Professor,
Ophthalmology and Visual Sciences
Professor of Internal Medicine,
University of Michigan Medical School,
Ann Arbor, MI

LIGHTNING IN A BOTTLE: TURNING SCIENCE INTO MEDICINE

"Top Ten Therapeutic Targets for NMO" were the audacious words Dr. Yeaman wrote across the top of a whiteboard on a warm March afternoon in 2010 on the second day of our Scientific Summit.

Therapeutic targets? That was pushing the envelope, for sure. Many in the room didn't yet fully understand the disease, let alone know how to treat it.

The Rose Story Farm—an old English country home close to our avocado ranch in the foothills above the seaside town of Carpinteria, California—had a clear view of the ocean to the west and the low mountain peaks to the east. And it had every ecosystem in between. This rare spot was a bit of heaven where I have done some of my best problem-solving. I had a hunch that if we hosted our own NMO Summit there and somehow got the best of our braintrust out of their labs and out of their elements for a brief window of time, maybe we could spark a rare "Eureka!" moment. Cures—like diseases—can strike when you least expect them, and there was nothing like changing the environment to nudge along a little serendipity.

Thirty of our leading researchers and a handful of expert advisors had just returned from a sunshine break and had taken their seats around a very large table that filled the room. I leaned in. Instead of continuing to review basic science as we had planned, I felt an extra surge of energy in the room and wanted to ask them to think about questions they might not have anticipated. My instincts told me this could be a way to encourage everyone to move away from preconceptions and prepared remarks in order to be bold, to challenge dogma.

"We're going to set aside the agenda—and shift your focus." With that I spread my hands wide, saying, "From here . . ." and then narrowed them, "to here." What I hoped we could do, I said, was to let go of the abstract brainstorming and focus on the key goal now written at the top of the whiteboard.

There was a silent pause in the room. Then the ideas began to flow. Dr. Scott Zamvil was among the first to speak, urging us to look at the importance of T cells in NMO. Then Dr. Jeff Bennett followed by talking about the understanding that B cells make the hallmark autoantibody NMO-IgG in the disease. Soon there were many voices chiming in, from bright young stars like Dr. Ben Greenberg to bold veterans like Dr. Alan Verkman, Dr. Larry Steinman, Dr. Vijay Kuchroo, and Dr. Vanda Lennon, who were all unafraid to question everything. Dr. Yeaman quickly began to connect the dots—diagramming in front of their eyes the pathways of an immune system puzzle that was revealing a picture of realistic drug targets. There was a magical give-and-take electricity in the room, and with each new suggestion, he would reply, "What else? Look at the connections."

More and more suggestions came. More and more limitations were overcome. Exciting new therapeutic concepts and targets emerged. Some of the targets could repurpose drugs already approved for other diseases. Others would require new drugs altogether—but that could quickly be tested for proof-of-concept in the laboratory and, if positive, could readily lead to clinical trials.

The session lasted more than four hours. As I listened and watched it unfold, I knew we were witnessing a pivotal moment in a revolution—when impossible gives way to possible. These were thirty of the world's leading voices in their respective arenas of science and medicine, all being challenged to open their minds and expand their limits of the known "pharmacopeia"— to consider everything in the medicine cabinet and across the disease spectrum. No suggestion was too radical or too obvious or too *anything*.

Dr. Yeaman conducted this like a symphony, at times promoting discussion and at others inspiring debate—all the while integrating each potential target and its location into the molecular mechanism of NMO taking form on the whiteboard. A key aspect of the process was to keep it focused on feasible, practical goals. Leading-edge treatments are great if safe and effective—but they will not help anyone if they cannot be readily accessed, produced, and administered. So in thinking about what targets would be most feasible to industry, we also talked about: 1) whether experts in the room had studied the target in any disease capacity—rare or not; 2) if any knew of experience of repurposed drugs with respect to potential application to NMO; 3) publications that could address the scientific rationale for a given clinical trial candidate; 4) the relevant intellectual property and patent landscape of the drug or candidate; and 5) how unconventional clinical trials, such as adaptive trial designs, might be used to speed these agents into the most meaningful real-time testing in NMO patients.

It's worth repeating one of the most important decisions we made as a foundation from day one: our choice to allow inventors and their institutions to retain all intellectual property rights—even if the discoveries and inventions were funded entirely by us. You might think these points would be themes we would *not* want to emphasize. There is a bias in assuming that patenting a great discovery is all about money. But profit and prestige are not the whole picture. The way I see it, the most driven researchers want to see their best ideas help countless patients.

The point that's often missed, as Dr. Yeaman has reminded us all, is, "Even the greatest discovery in the test tube will never become a drug in the clinic—will never help a single patient—*unless* it is patented." In fact, every drug candidate must have a plan for commercial investment and return on investment. No patent—no plan. After all, the cost of scientific and medical research for drug development is in the multimillions just to get to the clinic—and clinical trials cost even more. So there must be an investment motive. Business 101.

There was another wrinkle: the timing of patenting versus publication. One reality is that if publication occurs before a patent is filed, it can mean no possibility for a future patent. Yet patent applications can take time—and we wanted the world to know about breakthroughs as soon as possible. How did we overcome this dilemma?

Well, we planned for it and made sure we optimized timing in every way possible—relying on those advisors who had a rare combination of scientific and medical expertise *plus* proven experience in turning molecules into medicines. To name a few: Dr. Terry Blaschke and Dr. Terry Smith—or T1 and T2 as we respectfully referred to them—along with Nobel Prize winners Dr. Peter Agre (who discovered aquaporin-4 and like molecules), and Dr. Peter Doherty (who discovered how T cells recognize foreign versus self-antigen proteins), and a handful of other rare luminaries. And then there was Dr. Yeaman, whose acumen spanned immunology, drug discovery, and beyond. A leader among leaders, he was more or less a unicorn, even among these other rare experts.

All these strengths were brought to bear in that four-hour session

when everybody started chiming in about actual targets for new solutions to NMO. To me, it felt like the preceding century of Devic's disease
took a quantum step in evolution in one afternoon. We did not censor
or reject or qualify any suggestions—and we heard from everyone in the
room. Then and only then did we start to prioritize the list until we had
narrowed it to a "Top Ten."

I don't remember time passing. What I can recall is that suddenly
there was a moment when everyone looked up and there on the whiteboard was a drawing of the immune system and ten viable targets—for
which there were existing or realistically achievable drug candidates that
could improve the lives of NMO patients!

Some of the science was above my Dr. Mom capacity to grasp, but
my intuition picked up on the sparks of energy lighting up the room. We
might not have known it at the time, but these hours spent spitballing
ideas and refining them for the whiteboard had served as the incubator
for specific new drugs to treat NMO.

We caught lightning in a bottle—it was the birthplace of NMO clinical trials and creating our one-of-a-kind Industry Council.

CONCEPTS BECOME REALITIES

All of the top ten therapeutic targets discussed were promising for different
reasons. Three in particular leapt to the top because they involved *repurposing* drugs that were already approved for a disease other than NMO.

On its surface, the science of immunology-meets-medicine can seem
complex—even overwhelming. But to turn laboratory concepts into
life-saving realities, I had to keep learning. That meant getting up to speed,
even more, on how to speak the molecular and cellular language of NMO.

Once more, I turned to Dr. Yeaman, who I can always count on to
convey the Sanskrit of science into a simple story that every self-taught
Dr. Mom or Dr. Dad or Dr. Friend can grasp. Sometimes the imagery can
almost come to life, like a scene from a play.

For example, one of the first discussions that came up was about targeting B cells. These special white blood cells make antibodies—and if the NMO-IgG antibody really was the main culprit in the disease, targeting B cells made sense. To do so, drugs would need to target *only* B cells. This was the promise of precision medicine: target only the disease-causing cells in the body. Two key B cell markers are called CD19 and CD20. The drug Rituximab targets CD20, and now we were talking about using it to treat NMO. In one proof-of-concept study at the time, Rituximab helped some NMO patients avoid relapses. However, there were some patients who did not benefit. So an alternate idea was to focus on a therapeutic antibody in development that targeted CD19 on B cells. One thing led to another, and that thinking would ultimately spur one of the first formal clinical trials in NMO, testing anti-CD19.

The power of our incubator session paid off big.

For me to appreciate the synergy that had taken place, I had to learn even more lingo—and pay attention to the poetry of it too.

The Greek term *leuko* means "white," and the latin term *cyte* means "cell." Not so hard to figure out that "leukocyte" refers to white blood cells. Meanwhile, protein molecules most commonly end with the letters "in"—hemoglobin, insulin, albumin, and so on. So it was no surprise that the term "interleukin" referred to proteins that communicated between white blood cells.

Medspeak 101—check. This language added drama for my understanding of the NMO play.

"In a healthy immune response," Dr. Yeaman went on, "it is essential for leukocytes to know where to go and what to do. Interleukins provide some of the most important instructions from one white cell to another in defense against infection—or in causing a rare autoimmune disease."

Aha. Now I knew why everyone in the room was excited about another potential target for NMO therapy—interleukin 6, or IL-6.

Before I knew it, I was getting a dose of ancient Roman mythology and a reference to Janus, the god with two faces who presided over both war and peace. Inflammation also has two faces. On one face, IL-6 is required to protect against disease-causing microbes or even human cells that would otherwise cause cancer. On the other face—out-of-control inflammation led by IL-6 can kill a person faster than any cancer or infection. IL-6 is one of the master switches of inflammation and whether it targets self or nonself. I knew from earlier science we had funded: IL-6 seemed to play a key role in NMO.

A drug that calmed the IL-6 pathway? Of course. But wouldn't blocking an infinite number of IL-6 molecules be hard? Everyone in the room was on the same wavelength and focused on a new strategy—to target the receptor of IL-6 (IL-6R) on immune cells rather than the IL-6 molecule itself.

In my own mind, I thought of it this way: instead of trying to block an invisible cell phone signal that can go in every direction, block the *specific cell phones themselves* that can receive the signal. And because an IL-6R inhibitor was in development for use in rheumatoid arthritis, we would not have to reinvent the wheel. All we would have to do is get the company developing this new drug to understand the importance of testing it in NMO patients.

One more target that stirred a lot of buzz for testing in NMO was a molecule called C5.

I understood this was one of the proteins in blood that makes up the third rail of the immune system known as "complement." When NMO-IgG binds to AQP4 on astrocytes, it triggers complement proteins through a cascade. From inactive to active, leading to enhanced inflammation. In an autoimmune disease, that's a big problem. In this chain reaction, C5 amplifies inflammation in the optic nerve, spinal cord, and brain tissue in NMO.

My sense of urgency was escalated recalling that when Ali was first diagnosed, NMO was not known to damage the brain itself. Now we had learned that it could. Sobering? Absolutely.

But as good fortune would have it, a C5 inhibitor had been developed for a rare blood disease, and now there was a real possibility for clinical trials that could test its effectiveness in NMO.

In one afternoon of brainstorming, we had come up with three realistic and available possibilities to pursue right way as potential new treatments for NMO. Suddenly it seemed possible to get clinical trials in humans started in record time.

REALITY CHECKS AND BALANCES

Not wanting to lose a second of momentum, we emerged from that incubator meeting and began immediately to talk about outreach to industry. We could start by contacting executives at the pharmaceutical companies who already had the drugs that corresponded to the targets in NMO. Over the next two days, Dr. Yeaman took charge of masterminding a set of detailed one-page concept sheets of these three drugs and the other seven in our Top Ten—and then developed a ten-minute killer presentation showing my blueprint for how we built the Foundation to find solutions. A massive undertaking.

Reality checks can come in ways you might least expect. In our case, identifying promising drug candidates for a rare disease like NMO with such speed actually worked against us at first. Much to my surprise, after we started putting the word out to top-level people in the biotech and pharma sector, it took more than a year for them to actually *believe* what we had accomplished in such a short time—and then to get them to agree to a meeting. Was it really that tall of an order for a multibillion-dollar corporation or a regulatory agency to do things in a way they've never done before? Apparently so.

All I wanted was a chance to make the case about the benefits of trials for drugs they *already had approved* or had in development for other conditions. If the science made sense, why not look at these drugs in rare diseases like NMO? And even more than experts in immunology—I was ready to bring in a crack team of number crunchers to support my case.

Show them the math, show them the money.

Wearing my entrepreneur's hat, I knew the best way to get into the heads of industry executives was to let financial analysts review calculations about how profitable investment in rare could be.

And let me make a sidebar comment here to dispel a bit of an unfair label: Pharma executives can have hearts and want to see patients benefit. They have parents and spouses and children and friends and colleagues too—some of whom are affected by terrible diseases. But the message of investing in a rare disease would only be meaningful if rare could somehow be linked to common. And that is where our new insights into autoimmune disease shined: NMO was a model rare disease that could open new doors to treating or curing many more diseases.

To me, this was a no-brainer. If we had identified a target that would work with a repurposed drug that a certain pharma company already had—say, to treat cancer—and if we had already done the research demonstrating the scientific case to test it in NMO, and if solving NMO would offer a springboard to treating other autoimmune diseases, why wouldn't they want to get on board?

In the days of building my industry-changing cosmetics company—or Bill his infomercial and marketing empire—I never dreamed the skills and experience we were gaining would one day be key to curing a disease. The fact that Bill and I knew how to create business success and had applied those principles to running the Foundation gave us credibility with the pharma industry. They had an incentive for hearing us out.

There was another message too that I hoped would resonate.

It's true that pharmaceutical and biotech companies are in the business of making a profit. That's why opportunity was the name of the game. However, many companies who invest in therapies and cures are also in the ethical business of improving and saving lives. Some of their key executives have trained and worked at the higher echelons of the medical field as researchers and clinicians. Many we began to identify had come from prestigious careers in neurology and immunology. I had to believe they would value the promise of breakthroughs in NMO almost as much as us.

I had to believe in the heart connection. I had to take leaps of faith—that if I told our story they would care about our mission and draw from what brought them to their calling in the first place. I had to believe they also felt a moral responsibility to invest in a future in which there were no more medical orphans.

Why would it need to be one way or the other: profits or patients? Wasn't there a middle ground between industry's realistic expectation to do good for shareholders and our expectation for them to do good for the world? I believed there was.

But first we had to be heard, and that seemed like it was taking forever. After putting out feelers to everyone in industry and making little progress, I was encouraged when interest began to trickle in, finally, by the middle of 2011—starting with the decision makers at the very companies whose drugs matched our targets. The amazing drug concept sheets that came from our incubator session got their attention. So did the number crunchers I brought in to do the math and show in dollars and cents that their investing in NMO could be worth it—especially since we had already invested in the science. And I could feel in those conversations that heart mattered too.

But what made everything move forward was not us trying to sell them on running clinical trials. Nope, it was much more simple and much more real than that. I invited them to get to know us better and then see what they thought. No obligations to do trials, no barriers or requirements to having some sort of collaboration—unless that made sense for their goals too. We had always drawn the right collaborators our way by using a lot more carrots than sticks. The wins had to be mutual. Our message was just that we were putting it out there and looking for *partners* in solving NMO. We wanted them to win because if they did, there would be a safe, effective, and approved treatment for NMO. We wanted them to become part of our Industry Council.

It could have been nothing more than old-fashioned curiosity—wanting to seize an opportunity—or not wanting to be left behind. At least that's what it seemed at our Roundtable and Patient Day events in 2012 when we invited industry leaders from (what were at that point) competing companies to join us. And there would be more industry and government leaders to attend later events—and in greater and greater numbers.

Even though it had taken us longer than I'd hoped to get these potential new partners in the room, things were about to speed up exponentially.

Our blueprint strategy was at work: to get new partners to join in you had to show them the value proposition—in patient lives saved *and* market shares earned. That was more important than ever now that the mothership was prepared to jump to hyperspace—as we advanced closer to clinical trials.

PATIENT CONNECTIVITY

"Numbers don't lie."

Ali spoke that truth in making her opening remarks at our October 2012 Patient Day at that same historic moment when we had industry representatives in the room for the first time.

She recounted her medical experience over the past nearly five years: sixty doctors' visits, sixty-two sets of labs, thirty-two MRIs, fifty-two IV infusions, and sixteen full-blown attacks. Ali acknowledged that those numbers would *not* seem ridiculous or extreme to her fellow patients and their caregivers.

All my sorrow came flooding back.

No matter how many times you hear those numbers, it's impossible not to feel that stab in your heart, that turn in your stomach, that pain—for every patient—and that burning hope in your throat that you can and will make it better.

In those kinds of moments, you have to be present-focused, let go of the past, and put all your energy and attention on pushing the science onward to how to prevent future attacks.

Other numbers jumped to my mind—the dozens of pills that Ali and many NMO patients swallowed every day.

That's why I had to believe in the promise of new and improved treatments, of course. We were fighting the harsh reality that none of the drugs used to treat NMO were FDA-approved, because in trials they hadn't been proven to be both safe *and* effective. Most had side effects ranging from discomfort to risk of death—which was just not acceptable.

Amid those fears, I felt all the more strongly that if we could convince potential industry partners to work with us—and together with one another—for the first time in history, we would see testing of drugs specifically for NMO that could be approved if safe and effective. And . . . our studies of biomarkers in parallel with their experience in clinical trials could enable us to *predict* attacks and target the causal molecules or cells to intervene *before* they happened.

We had to do better—for NMO patients and every autoimmune patient. If we could only speed up the clock on drug development, we could change a lot of the bad numbers. With better treatments would come fewer daily pills . . . fewer relapses . . . fewer losses.

I desperately wanted us to find ways to avoid prolonged use of steroids—even to lower the dosages for maintenance that many autoimmune patients take as part of their daily regimen to control pain or ward off relapse. As our Patient Guide to NMO presented in bold print: "Steroids are powerful medicines that suppress the immune system overall, including the ability of the body to fight infection and promote wound healing. In addition, steroids can have other adverse side effects, such as weakening of the bones, predisposition to kidney stones or cataracts, and changes in metabolism, including fluid retention, increased blood pressure, or weight gain."

On the other hand, steroids could do the miraculous—quenching the fire of relapse inflammation, protecting against tissue damage and permanent disability. The problem was that they could suppress the immune system too well, leaving a patient vulnerable to infection or cancer they would not have gotten otherwise.

My concerns only intensified my will to collaborate with industry partners—especially now that there were new technologies in the works for precision targeting as an alternative to immune suppression. The new approach would be like using the most precise forceps as opposed to the biggest sledgehammer. I could vividly imagine the difference this kind of progress would make for Ali and all NMO patients—as well as the countless other patients freed from the risks of broad immune suppression. Those would be world-changing, revolutionary numbers.

There were other numbers to consider. In her remarks that morning, Ali went on to talk about her favorite: "One."

Her point was to remind everyone how patients and families had gone from feeling totally alone to becoming *one* NMO community and *one* family. She rallied all to remember how each of us had a role to play in understanding the disease, improving treatments, ultimately finding cures. Combined, each of the ones could erase all the scary, painful numbers in the world of NMO. It all mattered—donating blood and data and stories. Everyone taking action, all together. Those single acts would add up, and those numbers wouldn't lie either.

As Ali spoke, I glanced around the room and saw patients and caregivers nodding in agreement—inspired. Our patient connectivity was another reflection of the Power of Rare, and I know it had to be meaningful for our industry guests in the room.

The timing was great too.

This was during the same October week when *Saving Each Other* was hitting the bookstores, when we'd been making major media strides, and in the same period when we debuted the first edition of our Patient Guide, *NMO: What You Need to Know*. This was the resource, of course, that contained all the information I wished had been available to our family when Ali was diagnosed. (To date, we have gone back to print twice because of so many advances in NMO, and it has been published in an interactive digital format as well.) We had lots more to report this same month about how our International Clinical Consortium, Biorepository, and CIRCLES programs were swinging into full action and grabbing global attention.

This was Ali's second year to deliver opening remarks to the global NMO family, and to welcome all to a day focused on patients—our real heroes. The year before, she had asked everyone to imagine a world without NMO.

Ali later confessed to having been nervous speaking in front of everyone her first year (not that *anyone* would have guessed). This second year, she seemed like she'd been an advocate all her life—there to send a message of empowerment to her fellow patients and caregivers. Ali also added humor to the mix by thanking everyone for "giving me the chance to improve my public-speaking skills."

Ali, already a sophomore in college, had been organizing TEAM NMO for an upcoming Walk MS in Santa Barbara. She had recently begun putting out the word on Facebook about the importance of building bridges to other organizations and the public at large:

NMO is very similar to MS in terms of its presenting symptoms, and the two disorders are often confused for one another. Since NMO is such a rare diagnosis, fewer doctors are aware of the condition, and thus more patients with this disease are mistakenly diagnosed with MS. The purpose of Team NMO in this walk is not only to spread awareness about NMO, but also, more importantly, to give this disease a voice and let it be heard.

On top of everything else on her plate, Ali was helping MS patients as well as NMO patients. Not only that, but around the room I saw eyes lighting up and notes being made by those who wanted to get involved to help too.

And then I had a thought about how to further patient advocacy. Why not develop kits and tools for anyone in our community looking to become an advocate?

Putting together kits was a throwback to my former life, back when I did things like coming up with a learning kit for applying cosmetics and even an all-in-one makeup survival kit. An advocacy kit was totally in my wheelhouse.

My next note to self included assembling materials for kits such as patient resource guides, "Everything You Need to Know" NMO/MS brochures, interactive slide decks, and order forms for NMO share packages. We also could develop a "Start Your Own Support Group" tool kit, available online or in person for those who needed guidance connecting to patients in their areas.

Anyone who shows how an idea can be implemented or a vision can be turned into reality is a blueprinter. As a proud blueprinter, I could see that the patient connectivity was alive and thriving in our room. NMO patient support and chat groups were just starting to form—from NMO Parent Support Groups to chat groups for Teens and Young Adults with NMO. There was even a men's patient support group called NMO Bros. Regional in-person meet-ups were beginning to take place. Empowered patients had been taking steps to put together their own gatherings and even mini-conferences, sometimes with medical experts on hand and sometimes for social, fund-raising, and awareness efforts. We needed everyone to become blueprinters for the cure.

Now we needed the whole thing to go national, and then global.

What did all this have to do with clinical trials? As I saw it, our connection to potential industry partners would happen in the room between them—the ultimate sponsors of trials and the patients who stood to gain or lose the most based on the outcomes. These were the patients who would make the heroic choice to enroll in trials. Without that courage, none of the other opportunities mattered.

In our morning Q&A panels that brought together patients with clinicians, I was proud of how increasingly vocal NMO patients were in wanting to do more to contribute to better treatments and a cure. All who spoke had faced down a relapse and were eager to know when there would be alternatives to their current treatments and how they could play larger roles in educating others. Just as inspiring was how closely our panels of doctors and scientists were really listening to patients and their concerns.

Later, I heard comments from our industry guests about how much they had learned by hearing directly from patients. As a matter of fact, that process would lead to an idea for an unprecedented study of NMO patients—one that would be shaped and funded by our new partners coming together to collaborate as they had never done before.

Unheard of.

But true. Our blueprint had succeeded in bringing competitive pharma companies to the table, and had catalyzed a unique collaboration among them.

Yes, we laid the groundwork. The potential to pair our experts in science and medicine with their drugs and dollars and expertise was always there—but we didn't start from that framework. We started with the opportunities—the science and the numbers that didn't lie. And in the end it was empathy and connection to patients that ultimately sealed the deal for competitors to come on board as part of our Industry Council.

We invited every member of industry to join our council. And if we were to accelerate the entire pipeline from test tube to treatment, we knew we needed to get NMO on the radar screens of the agency partners as well. Having succeeded in their own research careers, our advisors had earned respect and connectivity from leading research institutions such as the National Institutes of Health and the Immune Tolerance Network. We also gained strong alliances with parallel organizations, such as the National Multiple Sclerosis Society, the National Organization for Rare Disorders (NORD), NeuroNEXT, and many other groups. And yes, we gained the attention and worked closely with the regulatory agencies: the US Food and Drug Administration (FDA), the European Medicines Agency (EMA), and the Pharmaceuticals and Medical Devices Agency (PMA) in Japan, to name a few.

The "impossible" part of this story wasn't getting competitors to sit down together to advise us on how to revolutionize the drug-development process for treating and curing a rare, mysterious, and complex disease. The part of the equation that was once inconceivable is how these competitors worked together and with us on leading-edge projects of life-saving benefit to NMO patients—and, really, everyone in the world.

The motivation might not be so mysterious.

It was about the opportunities to do the so-called impossible that were not to be missed. And it was about the fact that there was a blueprint in place for turning those opportunities into realities—a win-win for all.

That NMO is rare has inspired scientists, clinicians, advocates and industry to collaborate in elucidating disease mechanisms and addressing unmet medical needs of people living with the condition. The Guthy-Jackson Charitable Foundation's leadership is galvanizing and mobilizing an entire community of champions and is itself an inspiring achievement.

—Peter S. Chin, MD, MSJA
Group Medical Director, Neuroscience
Spectrum Medical Unit, USA Medical Affairs,
Genentech, San Francisco

PATIENTS PRESS THE "GO" BUTTON: NMOtion

By the end of 2013, as Bill and I reviewed our annual founders' letter, we both exhaled in a combination of relief and hope that we could now officially announce the next phase of our journey: industry-sponsored clinical trials.

Our incubator summit meeting three years earlier felt like a lifetime ago, although we had walked a direct line from those Top Ten targets on the whiteboard to the rightful industry sponsor. For starters, MedImmune would be testing their anti-CD19 drug, MEDI-551, to effectively deplete B cells—but in a more explicit way focused on NMO. As for the IL-6R inhibitor, Chugai would sponsor and launch two clinical trials of their drug, SA237—after a small study with this drug in Japan had shown a benefit in preventing relapses. Likewise, based on an open-label study that suggested its C5 inhibitor, eculizumab, could be effective in reducing NMO relapses, Alexion began a clinical trial as well. Meanwhile, other companies were in the wings planning trials of their drugs—all focused on NMO. Rare orphan disease that it was.

We had eliminated seven to ten years of development for clinical trials—and more were being primed. But our role did not stop there. It was up to our industry partners to conduct the labor-intensive clinical trials, but our advisors and experts aided their design. And, of course, it would be up to patients to learn about the trials and decide for themselves whether to join in or watch from the sideline.

And while all these huge advances fueled hope, for me they also created a new urgency to think and plan several steps down the road.

Questions had to be considered that I never had to think about during the time when industry hadn't responded to us. For example: How would we inform patients and doctors about the trials without showing preference for one trial over the other? How would patients have their concerns and questions met before even finding out if they qualified for trials? And of course the lines between personal privacy, healthcare, and clinical trials could not be crossed.

My first thought was that it was time to update and innovate with a new organizing and empowerment resource for our NMO community—parallel but distinct from our foundation website—that would usher in a fresh level of advocacy and action. We came up with a concept for an interactive website—a new NMO patient gateway—that was all about informing NMO patients of the many opportunities to participate in studies and trials now emerging. We called it NMOtion ("in motion"), capturing in one term the concepts of being NMO-focused and forward-moving. This user-friendly and interactive site was a one-stop shop, a patient-driven multimedia resource that connected to tools and guidance and included content about the upcoming industry-sponsored clinical trials.

As a foundation, we had to be completely neutral. Or as I always put it: "We are Switzerland."

Of course, we *do* endorse the concept of carefully designed and performed clinical trials as a best means to evaluate new or better ways to prevent, diagnose, treat, and potentially cure NMO. However, as a nonprofit charitable organization, we do *not* endorse any specific clinical trial, clinical trial design, agent, experimental drug or procedure, or pharmaceutical company. We do not participate in recruitment or eligibility evaluation for any trial. And we are not in any way involved in the performance, data assessment, interpretation, regulatory agency review, or recommendations that emerge from any clinical trial or its outcomes.

Our neutrality meant we had to fulfill a very challenging diplomatic role in the overall evolution of NMO clinical trials. Our role was to make objective information accessible and relatable to patients and their healthcare providers. Our responsibility was to promote informed decision-making, no matter what each patient ultimately decides for herself or himself. Patients pressing the "go" button—only if and when they were ready.

The vision to develop NMOtion included providing easy access to portals such as clinicialtrials.gov, a registry of detailed information on clinical trials for all diseases. But I also wanted to do something solely for NMO patients that gave them the freedom and transparency to explore all aspects of upcoming clinical drug trials. Two challenges arose in that process. First—how did we roll out NMOtion and make sure the global NMO community knew what it was all about? Second—how could we personalize questions about clinical trials to the concerns of patients, first and foremost? The answer to both those challenges came in the form of new films we created with the Wondros team.

The first, titled *Where Will the Cure Come From?*, was a starting point to let patients know about NMOtion and a call to action. It offered information and inspiration for patients to consider if they chose to participate in the CIRCLES study, and how each rare NMO patient held answers to unlock the secrets of NMO. The NMOtion dashboard offered everyone three simple steps if they chose to participate: Join, Donate, and Share. The visuals connected to the NMOtion gateway and the narration encouraged viewers to consider different ways they might be part of the cure: "Join a clinical trial—donate blood and data for research—tell us your NMO story. Today's actions hold tomorrow's cures. Together, we are in motion. Together, we are the cure." This is still one of the most inspirational pieces we have made, and many patients and doctors alike say they get goose bumps every time they see it.

The second film, *How Clinical Trials Work*, gave voice to patient questions and concerns. It addressed the basic logistics of clinical trials, from eligibility to enrollment to randomization, and yes even to the topic of placebo-controlled trials. But most important, it addressed among the most pressing of their questions—"When will I get better?"—and how clinical trials are designed to help answer that question. This film was scripted and shot as a conversation between an NMO patient and her doctor.

But that part was focused on the head. In this film, we also needed to be sensitive to the heart of NMO patients and their families. After looking at a lot of the videos online about clinical trials, I couldn't find any that addressed patient worries or were even told from a patient's point of view. So in the film, the patient expresses her desire for an alternative to the medications she has been taking—and then proceeds to discuss her fears about having an NMO relapse during the trial—being randomly assigned to the placebo group as opposed to receiving the new drug. In the video, her physician reviews the risks, explains how different patients may or may not be included in any given trial, based on their individual medical history, and how the process for selection works. He also goes over the safeguards and rapid response in the case of a relapse. He sums up with the keywords: "There are risks. It's going to be up to you to weigh the potential benefits versus the risks."

We felt it was of the greatest service to NMO patients to avoid any sugarcoating but rather to acknowledge this is a real disease and there are no guarantees. And that approach opened a door to seeing the sacrifice and nobility of NMO patients—and all patients—who participate in clinical trials. They are not simply serving themselves; they are serving all who share their disease and all who may be spared from doing so in the future.

In a sincere moment captured on film, the patient's honest yet courageous response is a way of reflecting what we had heard from patients all along: "Sorry, it just feels kind of lonely. I've been living with the risks of NMO for years now. I just want to get better. I want us all to."

After the doctor assures her, "That's what these clinical trials aim to do," the film concludes with her decision that she is ready to move forward—for herself and for all her fellow NMO patients. The visuals are full of light, nature, and possibility.

Out of all the videos we've created, this has become one of the most viewed and shared of our films—within and beyond the NMO community—because it addresses the many questions and uncertainties that inevitably come along with obtaining new and better treatments.

Once we had begun the conversation, we helped our industry council and the sponsors of the different trials go on to produce complementary educational webinars for all our stakeholders, including patients, caregivers, researchers, physicians, and other advocates. They also took up the reins and responsibility for outreach through social, digital, educational, and advocacy media to heighten awareness about clinical trials.

The more we achieved in partnership, the more our partners wanted to assist and contribute sponsorship to all our foundation events. We never required that, but as time went on, the Industry Council offered— and we said yes. In turn, we could focus our dollars on the mission-critical research and patient support. After all, clinical trials are all about transforming and saving the lives of fellow human beings who happen to have an unfair and unfortunate disease. And in the end—when all the dust settles and we look back on these revolutionary times—helping these people and their loved ones is what matters most.

Which brings me back to some of the lasting lessons learned in the experience:

- When it comes to valuing rare, perception can be a barrier. Look beyond the surface of stigma and fear to learn the greater truths to be found in the Power of Rare. The exception still proves the rule.

- Study the history of what you seek to change. There may be a reason why others have failed to revolutionize. Then look for ways you can do what they couldn't.

- Good ideas should never have to fall into any Valley of Death.

Learn to build bridges across them—in spite of those who say you can't.

- Whatever the undertaking, if you want others to listen and offer support—find their currency. It may be money—it may be heart. Deal in that currency and help them see how your work will benefit them.

- In forging partnerships, be willing to show them your hand, i.e., *your* blueprint. In our case, we let it be known that we were always searching to create revolutionary but fully synergistic teams. Everything we did had to have a life-saving, laser-focused purpose for improving the lives of patients—from molecular and cellular drug targets to information, tool kits, and videos for advocates to real-world clinical trials.

- Listen first. With us, hearing the views of industry and regulatory leaders before we asked for validation and support was an ace up our sleeve. We found common ground. Partnerships work for the betterment of all with shared goals.

- Always remember who matters most for your combined efforts. We held that patients and families are the mission and the cure. We were able to inspire partners who could understand *and* share the priority and purpose.

- Know that the journey can ascend faster than even you expected— so be prepared. Keep thinking big and beyond to prepare for opportunities, and learn to adapt to new challenges on the horizon.

Clinical trials? We didn't have the luxury for self-congratulation. Not until we had changed outcomes for patients for the better. Even so, we were on the move—on the threshold of the most exciting and promising chapter of our journey. We had formed brave new partnerships and were ready to ride the wave of an unprecedented convergence in science and medicine to go further than treatments—to address causes in order to effect cures. We could now focus on harnessing the healing power of the immune system itself.

I don't know if the optimists or the
pessimists are right.
But the optimists are going to
get something done.
—J. Craig Venter, PhD
Human genome pioneer now focused on
health longevity and personalized medicine.
Keynote Speaker 2017 GJCF International
Roundtable Conference

CHAPTER 7

THE RARE REVOLUTION

Picture this: It's midnight at the Los Angeles Convention Center, where 10,000 people have come to attend Tony Robbins's Unleash the Power Within two-day workshop. The attendees are deep in meditation as they prepare for the first night's activity of walking barefoot over a fifteen-foot gauntlet of hot coals. Among these 10,000 are one fearless, miraculous college graduate by the name of Ali Guthy and her almost fearless but still pumped-up mom—me.

Loved the meditation—but *walking on fire?* I wasn't so sure about that.

Tony and I had known each other since the early 1990s when we began to make names for ourselves in the infomercial industry. We'd been friends and colleagues ever since. I've always valued Tony's brilliant insights and empowering energy, which have helped in their own way in our journey to cure NMO. So when the opportunity came up to take part in the two-day event—including the firewalk—I figured, *Why not?*

Yes, my tootsies were a little tender and, of course, Ali's were fine. Even so, I would never want to trade the experience I shared with my daughter of being cheered on by Tony Robbins and 10,000 other people, all while inhaling and exhaling the power within that connects each of us to the universe. The instant you hit the coals, your senses soar—any doubts or distractions you may have had are replaced by a singular thought: *keep going*! We had to keep moving forward to the sound of thousands cheering, "Yes, yes, yes, yes!" There was no time to stop to question what made you decide to do something this bold. All you can do is say "Yes!"

In that midnight run, the past almost nine years flashed in front of my eyes. On launching our foundation, I knew we were taking on a bold and even audacious goal: curing a complex, rare, and dangerous disease. We were met with good days and tough days—we just had to keep moving forward. We were saying yes to facing fear and uncertainty and yes to hope, love, purpose, and the courage to move past limitations. And as I was saying yes to all that, I thought of challenges faced daily by every NMO patient like Ali—every caregiver and loved one. I thought of the daily firewalk that has to be taken by the most vulnerable among us.

As always, I asked myself what could be taken from that experience to share with everyone in our NMO community. Was there a metaphor for all of us that could be learned from running breathlessly over searing coals? Was the message, maybe, that the time had come to push further outside our comfort zones?

Or more to the point, I wanted to know how I could push myself and make sure my blueprint did more to capture the spirit of optimism that is our human birthright. How could we tap that force without ignoring the very real challenges, fears, and concerns of living with a disease that is itself a metaphor for uncertainty?

If ever there was a time to push past limitation, this was it. There were new, revolutionary technologies in medicine, science, engineering, data, design, and media that a few years before were only in the realm of science fiction. We were at the shoreline of the medical revolution of caring about rare and sharing solutions—a paradigm shift our efforts had helped make possible. We were on the verge of a new universal application of rare—of getting everybody in the whole world into the room to collaborate and accelerate advancements in treatments and cures.

We had lots of reasons for optimism and for believing we could magnetize solutions that have been hiding perhaps in plain sight. Or have yet to be found.

How could we translate that hope and belief into real breakthroughs?

Practically speaking, how do you make optimism a verb? Actually, that word is *optimize*. We had a multitude of resources and options we needed to optimize. We had to also look for new ways to prioritize so we could do things differently and more expediently.

How do you create a self-fulfilling prophecy from a firewalk to say yes and make it a key piece of your blueprint for change?

The question sends me back to a recent example of how hero patients in our NMO family have faced down the fear and uncertainty of their firewalks—and emerged on the other side as inspirations to us all.

The incident took place at a Patient Day event not long ago and in front of everyone in our packed ballroom overflowing with patients, caregivers, researchers, and industry leaders. It was one of those moments of truth that would leave a lasting and inspiring impression on everyone.

As Dr. Yeaman wrapped up the morning session, I watched him walking among the patients—and rolling up his mental sleeves to find a way to send them a message to reveal how rare and powerful they really are. He did a real-time back-of-the-envelope calculation of patient heroism. He began, "Consider this: of the three NMO clinical trials under way, on average each involves about 150 patients. If you put all of them together, there are about 450 patients around the world who are participating in clinical trials that have the chance to yield the first drugs ever proven to be safe and effective for NMO patients."

The room seemed to visibly brighten.

"In other words," he went on, "*a few hundred* rare and heroic NMO patients have chosen to do something that is likely to benefit the lives of *a thousand times more* NMO patients."

He was right. We owed this enormous debt of gratitude for every patient who didn't choose to have NMO but instead chose to do

something about it. That was the Power of Rare all right, making optimism a verb. We all stood to applaud every brave NMO patient who
each, in her or his own way, had chosen to walk the coals—past fear and
pain—so we could get that much closer to a cure.

We were all saving each other.

THINK SIMPLY, THEN BOLDLY

Whenever I've said we tend to make solving a complex disease harder
than it has to be, I've had to take a beat to explain myself. Clearly, there
isn't anything easy about curing NMO. My point is that sometimes, in
order to be bold, it helps to *think more simply* about the most complex
problems. Sometimes, even as you keep going, it can be a good thing
to push the pause button on the heavy lifting every once in a while and
allow yourself to see with fresh eyes and hear with fresh ears. Instead of
listening to fear, you tune in to the inner voice of your own intuition—the
voice of survival rooted in each of your cells.

For me, thinking more simply has often been about being able to step
outside the whole and look specifically at each of the moving parts to see
how to better integrate them. Call it streamlining or midcourse correction
or what you will, the NMO medscape was now in rapid evolution, and we
needed to evolve just as fast. The blueprint had planned for this, and that
new streamline gave us a sharper forward focus that could be communicated to everyone else.

Always looking for new ways to do that, I had a flash of awareness
after a couple of our first meetings with biotech companies—in the lands
of hoodies and brainy twenty-somethings who, in their spare time, were
creating crazy new blockbuster apps and start-ups for fun.

Apps? Hmmm.

Why didn't we have an app? The minute I brought it up, it turned
out our intrepid foundation team had been working on something already. We all agreed that although we'd developed some powerful resources for NMO patient advocacy—like our website and our NMOtion

gateway—we needed to make them more accessible. How could we simplify that ability to connect? How could we improve our advocacy tool kit by making information right there at everyone's fingertips 24/7? Within twenty minutes, we were ready to go. Yes, we were on it. We were making an app!

The NMO Resources app was fast-tracked for development and free download on all kinds of handheld devices. Our designers went above and beyond what I imagined could be possible, translating an encyclopedia's worth of information into simply organized sections such as *About NMO, Diagnosis, Videos, Events, Research, Clinical Trials, Advocate Resources, Blood Bank, and Find An Expert (Anywhere in the World).* There was also a *My NMO Notes* section we've been told has been life-changing—allowing patients to store and keep track of medical visits, test results, and past notes while also creating new notes and to-do lists. The app is continually being refreshed with up-to-the-minute breakthroughs—like access to the latest peer-reviewed NMO research papers, and new videos just added to our NMO TV link. Patients can join webinars for clinical trials at a moment's notice.

Also a part of our app is information about and links to other apps that can help improve a patient's daily life—like Dragon Dictation and Braille Tutor for sight-impaired patients, plus various medication tracker apps, the ORGENTEC Autoimmunity Guide (general information about autoimmune disease and lifestyle support options), and GI Monitor (for keeping track of, and info about, GI health and concerns). Plus, apps designed to bring more joy into daily life, whether by providing audio or digital books, guided meditations, or other ways to manage stress and promote well-being.

All of that arose from simple and bold thinking and from recognizing that we had to keep moving. We have to keep improving, adapting, and in some cases reinventing our resources—because doing so has directly and positively impacted the quality of life for patients and their caregivers.

Being bold doesn't always mean being radical or requiring an over-the-top result. It's about not being static or complacent—about never standing still. A lesson you definitely learn from running over hot coals.

APPRECIATE EVERY STEP OF PROGRESS

One simple truth about me is that I am a profoundly grateful woman. Gratitude has served me. And while I'm driven to finish things I start, I've learned that focusing so narrowly on a pathway goal can cause missed opportunities to see huge steps forward along the way. That's why, as we push this marathon ever onward and upward, it's been helpful for me to think simply by taking inventory of each mountain we've climbed—*before* taking on the next.

In less than nine years, there has been a total transformation in NMO science. We continually hear how unprecedented that is in the field of autoimmune research and possibly in medicine. The world has learned more about NMO in that time than what had been discovered in more than a century before. What was once a rare, incurable, and misunderstood disease—known in 2008 to only a few uber-specialists—is now being viewed as a solvable condition that has already spurred insights into other diseases. We have wired a global network connecting the leading academic and medical institutions around the globe. That connectivity has been our system for amplifying and accelerating the best and most cutting-edge ideas into actions.

By 2016, we had accomplished another "impossible" feat for a rare disease when, with our International Clinical Consortium (ICC), we aligned expertise from twenty-four countries to set new and uniform standards for NMO clinical research. We now had consensus guidelines for how researchers could collect and process biospecimens as well as access and share data in real time. In turn, our advisors were sparking new projects in the ICC based on a collective agenda that laid out the priority unanswered questions in NMO.

Our CIRCLES draw sites were also expanding daily, it seemed. By that same point we were already at sixteen clinical study centers in the

United States and Canada. With the recurring donations of blood and data from patients and controls, we had attained a wealth of new wisdom about NMO—with much more to learn as our longitudinal study continued to break new ground.

And in the middle of all this energy, my job was to continue to agitate, instigate, and motivate—whatever it took. Oh, and also to politely push to get us nearer to new functional remedies on the path to cures.

Three formal clinical trials were in full swing, and two more trials were moving closer to being ready. And another five were in the early proof-of-concept stage. And counting. By no surprise, in 2016 there were nearly fifteen industry leaders joining us for our annual Roundtable and Patient Day sessions. A year later there would be another twenty new names in attendance.

Meanwhile, our team was working with our Industry Council to refine clinical trial designs to best address NMO patient issues in the most custom and safe way possible. And regulatory agencies were now paying attention—listening and offering insights with respect to criteria that would be priorities for approval once trials had successfully been completed. That almost never happens. And yet, because we thought simply and just asked for guidance ahead of time, the agencies said yes to cooperating in ways that would streamline efforts down the road.

Our little rare disease was finally getting its due as we deepened our alliances with organizations like the Immune Tolerance Network (funded by the NIH) and NeuroNEXT. And thanks to a great working relationship with the National Multiple Sclerosis Society (NMSS), we even cofunded breakthrough science with them that provided new insights into both MS and NMO. We were always looking for ways to partner so that all we knew could be shared with others, and vice versa.

And the rare but mighty NMO was now on the political radar of Congress as a model of solving an autoimmune disease, thanks to California congresswoman Barbara Lee. She introduced legislation for funding NMO research, patient support, and further connectivity between private and public institutions to accelerate better therapies and a cure. Our growing numbers of unstoppable advocates had given voice to efforts leading to March being declared National NMO Awareness Month—with the vast majority of states saying yes.

Patients now had advocacy kits and could also receive training to do their own organizing, fund-raising, educational outreach, and awareness-building. Helping us to spread the word is our advocate consultant, Lisa McDaniel, who has dedicated her life to educating caregivers and patients alike as a way to honor the memory of her son, Collin. He was a little but fearless light in the darkness—who lost his struggle with NMO at age nine.

I often think back to those "whys" I scribbled over the pages of notes I made about the cruelty of NMO. We don't have the answers to why we lose patients, but what we do know is that for every parent and child, or family member or loved one, who are touched by NMO, we are that much more dedicated never to stop, never to give up.

Lisa regularly moderates teleconferences for patients eager to do more as advocates and is often an ear for those who want to do more but aren't sure how to begin. "The more there are of us," she often says to those who are nervous about putting themselves out there, "the wider the reach we have. It really is simple, though it may seem overwhelming at first. The hardest part is getting started."

And NMO patients are connecting in new ways too. Lisa has joined forces with Jesús Loreta—husband of NMO patient Maria—to host telecons for our caregiver support groups. Jesús and Maria attended our first Patient Day in 2009. At the time of her diagnosis, Maria had lost 90 percent of her vision and her first transverse myelitis attack confined her to a wheelchair. Eight years later, her health has improved dramatically. Her eyesight is restored almost completely, and she walks on her own. Recently, Jesús wrote in a blog update that the two of them had danced together in celebration of her progress.

My heart warms at this news—I appreciate every step forward for every patient.

Maria and Jesús are ambassadors of their message: "NMO may be part of our day-to-day now . . . but NMO is *not* our life!" In urging other

patients and caregivers to inform themselves and to start their own advocacy efforts, Jesús stresses the importance of asking questions and using
the resources made available by the Foundation. He has pointed out, "Any
new symptom is a new flag and a new question. Being informed helps
me to have the patience and the tranquility to overcome the fears and to
make the right decisions with Maria at the right time."

Beyond the support groups, more and more international and regional
conferences are being held—sometimes independently and at other times
with support from us and our Industry Council. In November 2016, the
First Annual NMO Conference for Patients and Healthcare Professionals was held in Los Angeles at Cedars-Sinai Medical Center.

By linking the event to the required continuing medical education
(CME) program, this was another way to grow physician awareness of
and commitment to NMO. We're able to benefit everyone involved.

In a moment of rare coincidence—or not—when I arrived at
Cedars-Sinai to attend the conference, I was informed by members of our
team that a young man had recently been admitted to the hospital—with
a new diagnosis of NMO. A dancer who had suffered a transverse myelitis
attack that had partially paralyzed him, he was fortunate that neurologists
on staff had been able to diagnosis him so quickly. The hospital brought him
down to the conference long enough for him to meet members of his new
family, and I'll never forget how he insisted on standing to give us all hugs.
Incredibly, he was cheering us on—promising to get involved as soon as he
was up and around again. That's what I mean by making optimism a verb.

While these kinds of programs don't always include patients, we're
always looking for opportunities to connect healthcare providers, industry
leaders, and patients in an academic setting to promote our CIRCLES
program and present the latest information about clinical trials. The effort
isn't ours alone anymore. Our blueprint for getting everyone in the room
is being applied in more and more settings that we don't have to organize
by ourselves or micromanage.

And there was never a better time for all of this outreach to catch
on—now that our work with the International Panel for NMO Diagnosis

(IPND) has meant that we have rewritten the book on NMO diagnosis. Not only have we improved the speed and accuracy in diagnosing NMO and related diseases, but we also validated our estimate that NMO is at least 50 percent more prevalent than previously known. The IPND's work has also helped our scientists and clinicians doing research so we not only know more precisely what NMO is—but also what it is NOT. All of this sheds even more light on its causes, effects, and clinical care.

Through all this progress, we were realizing that NMO was not as ultra-rare as once believed. The numbers over the years had grown from a few thousand to 12,000 tops—to 20,000 and then 35,000 after that. The latest estimate, that I repeat on purpose for impact, is that there may be hundreds of thousands of people in the world facing NMO. Were we trying to create a bunch more NMO cases? Of course not. But we wanted those who have NMO to know faster and get the right care sooner. The point is that NMO is everywhere—a global disease that, as Dr. Weinshenker observed—had for too long gone by different names. Not anymore.

As I took stock of all we had learned and achieved so far, I also confronted the fact that we had many more unanswered questions. The reality is that thinking simply doesn't change or simplify new challenges, discoveries, or information that may put earlier conclusions into question. For example, recent game-changing studies have found distinguishable forms of NMO. One of them, the more common that we've known since Ali's diagnosis, is referred to as "AQP4 positive"—which occurs in about 75 percent of NMO patients. These individuals test positive for the anti-AQP4 antibody (aka NMO IgG). Another form has been identified in some NMO patients who have tested negative for anti-AQP4. These patients have symptoms very much like classical NMO, but have autoantibodies to a different self-protein called MOG (myelin oligodendrocyte glycoprotein). Does this mean they are two separate rare diseases?

Many experts believe so, but the answer is that we don't know yet. What we do know is that this has pointed us in a powerful direction for forthcoming research. The more we learn, the better and more accurate our treatments will be, and the more these discoveries can be shared with investigators of other demyelinating and autoimmune diseases—like MS. These discoveries also tell us something we have suspected from the start: each case is unique—each *person* is unique. That's the rare revolution— bringing more pressing questions into the picture. Like—Why does the immune system react to AQP4 in one person, MOG in another person and maybe other proteins in others?

Our work was opening doors and chasing down answers.

Even while it's great to take a breath to see how far you've come, the next step is to take another, deeper breath and prepare to take your boldest action yet.

Victoria and Bill's philanthropy
and team-building skills serve as a
road map for how health professionals
have to reorganize and seek funding to
defeat rare "orphan" diseases
that neither government nor industry
are immediately interested in
studying, particularly in an
era of constrained governmental
support for research.

—Brian G. Weinshenker, MD

*Professor of Neurology,
Mayo Clinic, Rochester, MN*

SEEKING THE HEADWATERS OF CURE

More than anything, my practice of thinking simply has always returned me to *thinking urgently* to set priorities and act on them. We would be swift but never reckless. That's my version of optimism in practice and why, after the firewalk, I knew it was time to come up with a short list of revolutionary strategies and actions.

For starters, we were going to raise even our high-bar standard of "mission-critical" to research grant applications. If the science was compelling but didn't absolutely open up new avenues of understanding or move the dial closer to a treatment or cure, we would not fund that project. My mantra held: Lives were at stake and the clock was ticking. We were not doing esoteric research. Instead we would put more funding toward what we were calling Cures Workshops—with a focus on investing in the revolutionary science of tolerization.

There is a difference between a grant and an investment. In the past, we had actually granted funding to help explore repurposing potential new therapies for NMO, such as bevacizumab and cetirizine. Grants had also fueled a promising new therapeutic antibody that so specifically targeted aquaporin-4 that it was named aquaporumab. With this invention, Doctors Alan Verkman and Jeff Bennett have created a good antibody to compete with the disease-causing autoantibody NMO-IgG.

Investment was different. When we made the decision to invest in tolerization, this was a first for us—a private investment independent of the Foundation. It was not about profit but about perpetual motion toward a cure. Priming the pump. Investment begets return begets investment. We believed enough to provide these seed funds to spark clinical trials that would not have been done otherwise.

In simple terms, tolerization is the incredibly complicated process through which it could be possible to harness the power of one's own immune system to solve one's own autoimmune disease—permanently. If restoring immune tolerance to an NMO patient could be achieved, it would spare them from lifelong immune suppressive therapy which has undeniable risks.

Bill and I asked ourselves tough questions when the opportunity arose to partner with biotech and pharma companies entering the arena to begin turning the science of tolerization into medicine. *If not now, when? If not us, who?*

We said yes. From our earliest days whenever I heard about the basics of tolerization from doctors like Larry Steinman, Howard Weiner, Scott Zamvil, and Michael Yeaman—a process of fighting fire with fire to turn immune system poison into medicine—I sensed its potential for curing NMO and multiple other conditions. In effect, the approach can be thought of like an inverse vaccine: rather than turning up the immune response to a target, tolerization turns the immune response down to that target.

But simple as the premise seemed, we understood that assembling the means for applying the science and technology was anything but. *Except*—because of all the advances made in understanding NMO, plus a convergent surge in biotechnology that could allow engineering of the immune system—we now had a once-in-a-generation opportunity to apply the blueprint to tolerization for cures.

The reasoning was straightforward. From my first crash course in immune science, I could see how NMO was the poster child for what autoimmune disease is—a classic identity crisis.

Dr. Yeaman reminded me of the basics: "Every autoimmune disease, rare or not, suffers the same dysfunction—seeing some component of self as being foreign or abnormal." Or as *not* self. Autoimmune diseases are mistaken identity on a molecular and cellular level.

It turns out that for many (if not most) autoimmune diseases, that key component remains a mystery. Not so in NMO. As we'd known from the time Ali was diagnosed, in NMO that component of self that was being mistaken by the immune system as not self was the protein water channel, called Aquaporin-4.

"The basic goal of tolerizing in NMO," Dr. Yeaman explained, "is to reeducate the immune system to no longer mistake AQP4 as an enemy—but to reboot the system so that the mistaken identity would be no more."

As he'd pointed out before, the healthy immune system is the inner mentor that conveys the ultimate guidance to "know thyself."

Or, as Dr. Larry Steinman suggests in a short film I made on this subject: "Let's not tear down the whole immune system. Let's try to tolerize. In other words, shut off the immune system so only that one individual immune response is turned off."

Dr. Steinman had said years ago it would be possible to use advanced technology to prevent the attack on the AQP4 target in NMO and "then leave the rest of the immune system intact so it can fight infections like cancer and do what the immune system exists to do." Tolerization could be a twenty-first-century way to optimize the immune system—not minimize it.

A way to stop the horror of NMO *and* end long-term immune suppression? A mother's answered prayer. A prayer answered for millions.

A rare disease with a known target made it ideal, Dr. Steinman said, for pioneering the technology for what could become the "Holy Grail of antigen-specific tolerance." His belief was always that, "NMO represents the strongest possibility of showing proof of concept of this approach."

More and more, scientists and clinicians agreed.

How was this different from conventional therapies being tested in clinical trials?

A simple comparison was that instead of developing drugs to block the part of the immune system that is misbehaving in NMO, in tolerization you change the immune system.

"With tolerization," Dr. Yeaman explained, "the immune system is instructed to ignore—or just gets tired of responding to a specific target—and *stops* reacting to it. In short, the immune system becomes tolerant of that target."

I got it—if you expose the immune system to what had been the self-trigger—*but* in a way that induced a calming response—you could broker *tolerance*. Not so different from the way a vaccine works, just backward. In essence, *the cause becomes the cure.*

In NMO, the important role of AQP4 autoimmunity is well recognized and helps bring focus to research into etiology and therapy. Many other autoimmune diseases lack an analogous cornerstone, but can nevertheless extrapolate from the NMO experience to look for parallel mechanisms that guide research efforts. In this sense, NMO is a leader, as well as an example, of an important shift towards early use of potent targeted therapeutics.

—Gerald T. Nepom, MD, PhD

Maybe we could turn poison into medicine. My heart and my head agreed.

And our investigators have begun to decode a key aspect in the identity crisis—immune system checkpoints—which are the gateways of the immune system, where the difference between self and *not* self is tested. By analogy, these checkpoints might be equated to a bar exam for immune system cells: only those that pass the test are put on the job. On the one hand, you want the immune system to react to germs and cancer cells that the immune system sees as foreign. On the other hand, you do not want the immune system to react to normal, healthy tissues.

Putting all the experts' voices together—and adding that part of my own intuition to the mix—Dr. Yeaman underscored how this was bigger than one condition. "The more NMO can lead us to decipher the fundamental secrets of such checkpoints," he said, "the more we can use tolerization to cure NMO—and beyond."

This was the revolution.

He continued, "The ability to remediate, reeducate, and reboot the immune system will impact every aspect of health and well-being in the coming decades."

MARKING A NEW DAY IN NMO

As someone who has learned to speak science to understand how it will save and improve lives, I have to confess that reading scientific publications is sometimes a struggle.

There, I said it. It's true.

But in certain instances, I get really excited about the poetry of breakthrough science and don't want to miss a word.

That's what happened in September 2016—when a hallmark event occurred in the history of NMO. The prestigious journal *Neurology: Neuroimmunology & Neuroinflammation* published two groundbreaking papers as a two-part series titled *Restoring Immune Tolerance in Neuromyelitis Optica*. The papers were the result of two years of bold thinking by an extraordinary group of our advisors and innovators—each working within and beyond the boundaries of NMO.

Both papers broke the news to the medical world about all we had learned that could be applied to tolerization in NMO, and in some cases had already begun or was on the launch pad of clinical trials. Approaches included DNA vaccination and T cell vaccination, along with a sizable list of more complex molecular and cellular engineering methods already under intense study.

With the work at hand, the authors stated, "Advances in treatment could benefit individuals with NMO/SD and other autoimmune diseases, including arresting disease progression, prolonging intervals to remission, enabling tissue repair, and ultimately avoiding chronic immunosuppressive therapy." In short, cures.

The publications coincided with the launch of Phase V of our mission—Onward to Cures. Timing being everything, the two-part road map laid out the key immune mechanisms in NMO with potential for "therapeutic restoration of immune tolerance" and how tolerance-restoring techniques might be applied to patients.

According to the authors, "In theory, the identification of aquaporin-4 as the dominant autoantigen makes NMO/SD an ideal candidate for the development of tolerizing therapies or cures for this increasingly recognized disease." NMO really was the little disease that could.

Beyond theory, the papers went on to point out recent technical leaps in tolerization that had already been achieved in experimental models and, more important, were beginning to be tested in humans. Special focus was given to the regulatory T cells—responsible for applying the brakes on immune responses as needed—as well as regulatory B cells—along with new approaches to oral tolerization.

The compass provided by these papers was also our team's way of saying to others in autoimmune research and across the medical universe— *This is how it can be done to move ideas into clinical trials. And we want everyone to benefit and pursue new solutions made possible through new knowledge and emerging technologies.*

When I read both articles, I was encouraged. This wasn't *one* day or *some* day. These were specific steps we'd already started to take.

The language was rare and brave—reflected in the last line of the concluding paragraph: "Each of these perspectives is intended to shine new light on *potential cures* for NMO/SD and other autoimmune diseases, while sparing normal host defense mechanisms."

We were saying the word *cure* because this was what *tolerance* meant: heal the immune system and allow tissues chronically injured by inflammation to regenerate. We would soon be sparking clinical trials for tolerizing therapies that could heal the immune system. The era of antigen-specific medicine had begun, and we were at the forefront of it. Rare NMO was that canary in the coal mine getting everyone to pay attention.

Curing NMO through immune health could be reflected in the mirror of much more common diseases. We were applying insights learned from the newest solutions for cancer, transplantation, and infection to advance autoimmune science—and then turning it back to show that curing NMO would open doors of cure for those same millions of patients.

Common and rare. In this together.

The lesson of the firewalk continued to echo for me. Everything we did had to have a consequence—and there was no one road to whatever was going to be the Holy Grail for a cure. *Every* road counted, as long as it was heading to our true north.

The therapies for NMO that we already had coming through the pipeline had nudged us closer to the reality of tolerization. And as tolerization gained traction, we would go further—to gene editing to correct misbehaving DNA, and stem cell therapies to repair spinal cord, optic nerve, and even brain tissue injured by NMO. For real cures, it would not be enough to stop the disease in its tracks—lives needed to be restored to health.

So we weren't stopping at putting out the fire. We were also making headway with new allies in the science and technology of regeneration and remyelination—with cell-based therapies that could repair damage to the central nervous system. Early in our journey, in fact, my wonderful friend Sherry Lansing—a member of the board of directors of the California Institute for Regenerative Medicine (CIRM)—had invited me to present the NMO story to that organization and how our foundation was going to rewrite it. After telling my personal journey as Dr. Mom, I brought Doctors Ben Greenberg and Michael Yeaman up to share the podium with me to explain how stem cells could be retaught to tolerate AQP4, repair the myelin insulation on neurons that had been stripped away, and more. A short time later, in connection to this new association with CIRM, I was honored by being asked to sit on the board of UCLA Health System.

Our conversation about stem cells first took place in 2010, back when we had just begun to build our cure machine. By early 2016, the entire field of regenerative medicine had advanced so much that Pope Francis and the Pontifical Council for Culture had joined with world leaders and the foremost names in philanthropy, faith, medicine, and technology to envision a pathway for bringing cellular cures to those in need. That conference, to be held in the halls of Vatican City in April 2016, was where I had been invited to speak and share our NMO breakthroughs— and where Ali would be honored with a Pontifical Hero Award. When I shared that news at Patient Day, I could have sworn by the resounding applause that everyone in the room felt they would be attending right along with me.

And there was more, I continued. Besides the new dawn for possibilities of cures for NMO in stem cells, we were ahead of the curve in the fields of Big Data and supercomputing. Those visits to Silicon Valley had paid off—and we would soon be partnering with Google's Verily Life Sciences and others to drive an ambitious new biomarker project. Knowing biomarkers in NMO had given us clues to their involvement in the disease, and now we had begun to tune that knowledge to detect warning signs of relapses before they happened. We were on the move, hot coals and all. Once we solved these most upstream of all mysteries, we could prevent relapses before they began and, after that, NMO itself.

And the next firewalk was going to be translating all these very real capabilities into saving and liberating human lives. No, we were not at the cure yet, but at long, long last it was in sight.

That much I knew, just as I felt the sheer enormity of all who were counting on us to make change happen. The message of movement rang in my ears: "Keep going."

There was no other way. And yet, not all roads lead to Rome—as I was soon to learn.

THE RARE REVOLUTION

If it sounds like I've made it through unscathed after every firewalk I've ever undertaken, that would not be true. In April 2016, in the weeks and days leading up to our departure for the Vatican, I found myself being pulled down to the depths of a ferocious undertow of anxiety I had otherwise managed to keep at bay for many years.

Everything about the conference was a gift—from the opportunity to meet Vice President Joe Biden and hear about his Moonshot to Cure Cancer to the chance to share our innovative ideas about immunotherapy with philanthropist Sean Parker. And I mean, oh, my God—What else can I say?—the once-in-a-lifetime moment of having an audience with Pope Francis. How could I have ever dreamt that? More than anything, the prospect of attending the Pontifical Hero award ceremony for Ali would be marking the miracle of all the odds she had defied. Even just the opportunity to be in the mix of a world-changing conversation about how science, technology, information, and communication could positively impact human lives—it would be a chance to learn so much that would inform our rare revolution even more, and to share our blueprint for health.

I kept thinking about how a little more than eight years earlier I was lying on the floor frozen by anguish for my daughter and fearing the absolute worst—and never in my craziest hopes could I have predicted being asked to carry our road map for curing a rare, devastating disease like NMO to the Vatican. What a validation. The universe had tapped me on the shoulder and I had said yes.

Then why was I being taunted by anxieties I'd mostly set aside long ago? Was it the lofty magnitude of it all? Was there something in me that didn't feel like I had done enough to achieve an absolute cure—even with all the lives our collective efforts had saved and improved? Was I forgetting my knowledge of the immune system—that I had to know myself and my strengths? And my limitations? Was it a relapse of the fear of flying I thought had been banished after Ali's diagnosis—because I had no choice other than to get on those airplanes and travel to where our work could make the biggest difference? Was there some faulty wiring and messaging that made me worry somehow that this conference would take my eye off the ball?

Or was it much simpler? Was it just that I was exhausted and that making this trip had just landed on top of having done too much for too long without cutting myself some slack? Whatever the answer, I had to face down the reality of my fears and accept that I couldn't do it all. Yes, I was not immune, and this trip was a bridge—or a road to Rome—too far. At the last minute, I canceled, knowing we would be represented by allies in attendance. Still, the huge disappointment I felt in myself would be mine to shoulder.

That's the other lesson of the firewalk. While you must keep moving, it is also necessary to accept that not every gauntlet filled with burning coal has your name on it. You can't do it all and be in all places at all times—no matter how much you'd love to try. As apologetic as I was, Ali insisted that she could better spend her energy on climbing her next mountaintop—studying for her LSAT exam and beginning the process of applying to law school. Was she just trying to make me feel better? I don't know. The fact is—she did.

Even so, the biggest lesson from not going to the Vatican was that I would have to turn the energy of my own disappointment into even more lessons and more enlightened actions. Life is real, and none of us are perfect mortals. In the power of my own rare properties, those rare fears are still part of who I am—part of what drives me to be better. There was also the reality that whatever presents itself as the opportunity of a lifetime, no such thing really exists—it was an opportunity in that *moment* of a lifetime. There is always more opportunity to be found if you seek it.

Being real with myself when the dust settled soon had me back on my feet. And out of that process came a new vision for where we were headed next.

For most of our history—before writing this book—I avoided tooting our horn or talking too much about our blueprint. And I certainly did not want to suggest we were stirring up a revolution. My philosophy was always just to get at it, do the work that needed to be done, and prove to all of us that it was possible and doable. Then, and only then—once we'd achieved benchmarks to prove there was no such thing as impossible in NMO—then I believed it would be helpful to shine the light on our model.

So when I started to hear that other foundations, organizations, and even government programs were seeking out aspects of our blueprint to use in their work, I felt proud and honored. And then, as the universe so often does, just as I was asking myself how I could do more, I received a message of extraordinary validation from the National Women's Hall of Fame at Seneca Falls—I had been selected as a 2017 inductee.

Alongside nine other inductees—including Sherry Lansing, Temple Grandin, Alice Waters, and more iconic women trailblazers—I would be joining the rarest of sisterhoods. How had this happened? As I read the press release, I was humbled by their words:

> When her daughter was diagnosed with the rare autoimmune disease, neuromyelitis optica, (NMO), innovative cosmetics entrepreneur Victoria Jackson dramatically shifted her focus, talents and financial resources "from mascara to medicine." In the course of creating, funding and leading a research foundation, Ms. Jackson has shaped a paradigm-breaking approach to medical research. In

addition to connecting hundreds of innovative problem solvers from 28 countries and even more diverse fields of expertise in an unprecedented model of collaboration, Victoria Jackson has established a global network of patients, advocates, and healthcare stakeholders—with significant positive impact on the treatment of autoimmune and related diseases. Underscoring the transformative significance of Jackson's contributions, she is the recipient of multiple awards and is a passionate advocate for women's empowerment and entrepreneurship.

There at Seneca Falls, the birthplace of the 1848 launch of the modern women's movement, I would have the privilege of being inducted into the Hall of Fame, joining the 266 past inductees—women who for the last fifty years have been the pioneers, change agents, and revolutionaries who have transformed the world for the better.

So I suppose that even though all roads don't lead to Rome, they just might lead to somewhere else—like Seneca Falls. What matters is that you pave your own road to that place with the passion of something you believe in with your heart and your soul—to create new and better and rare for the world.

And those lessons have encouraged me to do more to share our blueprint. Not because I think we should have credit—that never mattered. The blueprint is a way to pay it forward by inspiring and informing others how we can all do more than we know to create change—in medicine and beyond.

What also matters is that the rare revolution is here, and we all have a responsibility to participate—and in time to make a difference. The door that leads to desperately needed answers will not be open forever.

We are all in this together, and every single one of us has a role to play in it.

The revolution has been built from many rare efforts devoted to world-changing causes that affect the health and disease—life and death—of every person on the planet. All 7 billion of us. The rare-inspired medical revolution will rise or fall depending on how we seize the moment. We have an unprecedented opportunity to take advantage of twenty-first-century cures that are just beyond the reach of our fingertips. We have to reach together. And so, yes, there is great reason for optimism and even greater reason to turn that optimism into your own daily action verb.

My blueprint going forward reflects a vision for even greater connectivity among all of the moving pieces that will get us to personalized and precision medicine for all. Our advances are driven by the most meaningful connections—between patients and doctors, between investigators and industry and regulators, and between leaders in all sectors of society who have the new opportunity to cooperate in converting vast storehouses of data into wisdom—and wisdom into practice.

The rare revolution rests on the shoulders of each and every one of us who cares about the future for every single one of us. We all have to take action.

You may be wondering how you can choose to begin or how to keep going when that part gets tough. Here are some lessons I have gained that may help:

- *Own your rare.* Know and cherish what makes you unique. But also know the universal truth as well—only by knowing rare do we know common.

- Like the message of the immune system, which teaches, above all, "know thyself"—the guardian rules for your health and well-being are in you. Look within to know the role you can play in finding cures.

- Be willing to adapt your blueprint for change. Accept the reality that you cannot do it all, and give yourself permission to learn and quickly get back on the road to success.

- Whatever your role—patient, caregiver, researcher, industry leader, regulatory agent, philanthropist, or as an ally in any important cause—know it's not just about you. You can ease someone else's burden by cheering them on as they travel their own roads.

- In the metaphoric firewalk each of us faces every day, don't be afraid to call the pain of walking over hot coals for what it is—pain! But also know that your struggles matter. Because they do. On a life-and-death road, they matter to us all.

By choosing to act even in the most challenging of circumstances, you flip on the switch of active optimism that is part of the voltage needed for any kind of revolution.

The other part of this massive energizing and organizing force is what I want to talk about next—and why it matters now more than ever.

Rare is the window into the unknown.

—Dr. Maria Spiropulu

In her Power of Rare 2017 Keynote
at the 9th Annual Guthy-Jackson Charitable
Foundation NMO Roundtable.
World-renowned experimental particle
physicist at the California Institute of Technology.
Member of the CMS collaboration at the Large Hadron Collider
where the Higgs boson Particle ("The God Particle")
was discovered in 2012.

CHAPTER 8

NO ONE IS IMMUNE

"Cancer."

The word stuck in my ears before I could comprehend what it meant. A wave of denial crashed upon the rocks of this reality. But the unchangeable truth that followed next couldn't be washed away: no one is immune.

All at once an onslaught of my worst fears began to overwhelm me. Like every parent, every caregiver, every change agent who commits to leading a journey to a better place, the sudden prospect of not being here . . .

Not being here for everyone who is depending on me? No, this can't be.

But it was more than a possibility.

It was a balmy Southern California day in late January 2014—not a cloud in the sky. A short time earlier, I'd been in my den catching up on paperwork and sitting on my favorite couch when I received a phone call from my doctor. He wanted to come to the house to talk to me in person about the results of a recent biopsy.

Wait. *What?*

Days before he had assured me that the chances of it being anything other than benign were less than 1% . That hadn't exactly made me feel better. Had my Rule of 2% suddenly been cut in half? I tried not to worry.

But as soon as I heard the doctor was making a house call, I was 99% sure that the news wasn't good. The shellshock of getting Ali's diagnosis had never left me.

As I built up an arsenal of illogical reasons why there had to be a mistake—sound familiar?—a logical thought crossed my mind. Somehow I knew that if it was bad news, the last place I wanted to get it would be sitting on my favorite couch—which would forever after be associated with cancer. If this was going to be a dark memory, I decided it would be best to be outside in the sunshine, and to have the doctor join me there. As if somehow sitting in a quiet garden on a pretty winter's day could change whatever he had to say.

But as I already knew, not every situation can be so spiritually controlled.

When my doctor arrived, the first thing he asked was, "Why are we meeting outside?"

I had to tell him the reason and admit that I anticipated the biopsy came back positive—and that I was in the 1% after all. He nodded thoughtfully and reassured me that I would be all right.

Still, when he uttered the word *cancer*—and then added that he wanted to schedule surgery immediately—I had to resist the urge to bolt again from where I was. Nothing made sense in that moment.

After I got past the shock, denial, and grief that comes with the truth that no one is immune, I began the emotional process of reaching out to family and friends. Ali tried to be stoic, and I did make her laugh about my couch story. All I could do was reassure her—and myself.

On the evening before the surgery, a group of my closest girlfriends—along with Ali, who had driven down from UCSB to be at my side—gathered quietly in my den and formed a healing circle of love and support around me. A large beautiful stone made of rose quartz was passed around the circle. As each friend took the stone into her hands, she would tell a personal story of some kind of challenge in her life and then metaphysically put into the stone whatever capacity it was that had helped her to heal.

In tears and gratitude, I listened to the stories, blessings, and prayers that each woman shared. One told her own story of overcoming the odds of a cancer diagnosis and put "humor" into the stone. Another recalled struggles as a single mom and put the discovery of "strength" into the stone. There were blessings put into the stone backed by recollections of faith and recovery. Then, at the very last—there was Ali—who held the rose quartz stone in her hand and took a breath before she offered up the rarest of all contributions.

"Mom," Ali began, "I've thought a lot about what else needs to go into the stone." And the more she thought about it, she said, the more she realized I was the one who was healing others and making sure that all would be well for them.

There were murmurs of agreement around the circle.

"And so," Ali announced, "I'm going to put *you* into the stone. Because that way I know you're absolutely going to be fine and you'll make sure that all will be well for you."

This was such a clear metaphor of our journey of *Saving Each Other*. Ali was saving me, again, not only from fear but even more by empowering me to know that all would be well—by putting me into the stone so I could do for myself what I did for others.

With that, she handed me the stone and I held it in my hands, pressed it to my heart, and refused to let it go for longer than a few minutes here and there until I fell asleep later that night. And when I went to the hospital the next day—with Ali and the rest of the family with me—the healing stone came on the journey too, along with all the prayers and blessings and me that had been put into it.

This was not, of course, the end of the story. And it was not the only instance of the lesson I can recall of realizing that no one is immune.

If the history of medicine is told through
the stories of doctors, it is because their
contributions stand in place of the more
substantive heroism of their patients.

—Siddhartha Mukherjee, MD, DPhil
Author, *The Emperor of All Maladies:
A Biography of Cancer*

TRUE STORIES OF HOPE OVER FEAR

I had spent all these years putting myself in patients' shoes. Though I had long understood that none of us is immune to being struck by a sudden diagnosis, I had lived that reality as a patient and now a survivor. I felt the need—more than ever—to do all I could to give back.

The world had become a much smaller place for all of us in the NMO family. Connected by a rare diagnosis, we grew that much closer—that much more knowledgeable of what it was like for patients and caregivers around the globe. Wherever patients came from—all across the United States and Canada or from overseas nations such as England, Colombia, Mexico, Belgium, Germany, Australia, South Africa, China, and beyond—we never seemed to have a language barrier. It continued to amaze me that out of all the people they knew before coming to Patient Day, most had never met anyone who shared their diagnosis. Yet from the instant they gathered in the room together, everyone was related. All ages, all backgrounds—the rarest of friendships—for life.

I'm still always struck by the question of what's going on inside and outside every NMO patient that connects each of them and results in the same diagnosis. Maybe it means the combination lock of this disease has many rare solutions. Or maybe it means there is an even rarer master switch that malfunctions in the innermost immune system core of every autoimmune disease. If we knew these answers, I keep wondering, would we not be that much closer to solving NMO? For clues to that mystery, we had to listen even more closely to patients.

Their stories are unforgettable. In my view, there is nothing more powerful than a true story—and nothing more meaningful than a rare story. That was one of the main reasons we set out to conduct a different kind of survey of patients and their quality of life. We had heard from patients over the years that feeling connected to a community and not being isolated with a scary diagnosis had improved their quality of life. We had heard how patients felt better and more empowered by taking an active role in a cause that mattered to everyone—and to themselves. However, this survey was the first time patients had been given the chance to tell their own stories in depth—aside from clinical data alone.

At our 2017 International NMO Conference—themed the Power of Rare—Ali, diagnosed at fourteen and now almost twenty-four years old, would be making a presentation at the Roundtable scientific sessions. This would be her first time doing so. She and a panel of fellow patients would join with scientists and clinicians and industry leaders to present the findings of this groundbreaking survey.

In designing the survey, we understood that everyone in the room would be able to really listen—to learn so much more about how to care for the person with NMO—not just treat the disease of NMO. Each volunteer patient had the freedom to describe her or his own personal views—with anguish or exasperation and every emotion in between—in facing the challenges required of living day to day with NMO.

The questions collected from 200 participants spanned topics from life and livelihood. Patients reported ups and downs (often in heartwrenching terms) in every aspect of their experiences—from physical and emotional health to the economic impact of the disease.

At the appointed hour in the early afternoon of our second day of scientific sessions, Ali went to the podium and was soon joined by several fellow patients. A hush fell over the room as we watched the participants take the stage—some in wheelchairs or with caregivers leading them to their spot, others appearing to be at the peak of health. The silence was broken as each storytelling hero began to express her or his hopes or fears.

Watching and listening, I was all the more inspired as each rare patient bravely rose to be heard.

A thoughtful woman who had struggled with NMO for years said with sincerity, "I am worried that my condition will worsen to the point that I will become a burden to my family—physically, financially, and emotionally. I do not want to be alone, but I do not want to be a burden to them or to anyone."

A young person recently diagnosed with NMO went on, "NMO patients such as myself are very hopeful that dedicated researchers will find causes and cures for NMO—through increased and sustainable funding for research and development. We can all spread the word and help educate the world about NMO and how we are solving it together."

And the Power of Rare was spoken through the words of a devoted partner: "As the husband of an NMO patient, I have seen how clinical trials are moving forward faster than ever. I have seen how the NMO community has been there for us. You guys are better than any medicine. I have seen improvements in my wife's quality of life. We now dance together again. And we have great hope for breakthroughs to come."

For some there was a shared concern. One patient, who was overwhelmed for many reasons, admitted, "It's harder to be hopeful when clinical trials can take such a long time and require so much effort that it's difficult for me to participate. I want to help myself and other patients, but I'm concerned that it is too much for me to do."

And the fear of being overlooked was evident in the voice of another patient, who said, "I worry that too few researchers are focused on solving NMO, and those who are will lose interest, energy, or funding to conquer this rare disease. Researchers, companies, and regulatory agencies must better coordinate to push development of safe and effective treatment more quickly for patients."

Another patient explained how the choice was made to move past fear and participate in clinical trials: "First, because I am very hopeful that new drugs will be safe and effective for me. And second, because I know that once there is an approved drug, many patients will benefit."

Several patients expressed gratitude to all the problem solvers. As one young patient put it: "I am grateful and my family is grateful for all of the work being done to help patients like me. All of the great hearts and minds working together give me sincere hope that I can have a happy and full life with my family."

This is the wish of so many patients with a chronic or debilitating disease—safer and better treatments, fewer risks in drug trials, new ways to prevent attacks, and a date certain for a real cure—to have the chance to live each day joyfully and boldly.

As Ali reviewed the main findings of the survey, she pointed out that, as a whole, NMO patients were more hopeful than they were fearful. Of course, there were concerns and fears—and these were serious. Yet despite the risks of relapses and treatments, hope was conquering fear.

This same presentation would take place again at the end of Patient Day. Fittingly, voices of patients and caregivers would be raised loud and clear to make their stories matter most toward finding a cure as a poignant close to the conference and plea for the future. The emotion in the room was even more resounding as every patient and caregiver in the room saw and heard their stories reflected in the voices of others. When Ali started to summarize the numbers and comments in the survey, she added another thought.

"As we look at concern versus hope and what it means for our quality of life and for our families," she began, "the question then becomes—how can we move the dial so that hope outweighs fear ten times over—so that we can all put our concerns and fears to bed?" She was challenging everyone to turn hope into a realistic end to NMO. Less a question than a statement, Ali added, "So we can live every day feeling better, growing stronger, and thriving in every way."

Ali was pointing to what I had always believed—that every patient is a miracle—putting themselves into their own healing stones, choosing each in their own ways how to be part of the cure.

Looking around the room, I spotted familiar faces of patients who had been with us every year since our first Patient Day and some who were new to us. Rather than seeing the room exactly, I felt the room. That was my old habit of putting myself in everyone else's shoes and trying to experience what they were feeling. I was in awe of each one of them—for their courage and for showing up. For giving me strength. They were my infusion.

Ali continued, speaking for herself and for other patients who had shared their stories and their truths. And here was her truth: "I firmly believe from the bottom of my heart that we are on the cusp of making leaps and bounds in discovering better treatments for NMO. And this survey shows that hope for finding a cure for NMO is alive and well and strong." Two of the patients seated on the panel stood up to applaud. More patients and family members followed from their seats. Ali spoke to the whole room as she went on. "We all know it's coming. How long? We know that if it's weeks, months, years—it's coming—it's going to happen. The minds in this room are going to make it possible."

Ali pointed to the doctors and scientists and members of the Foundation and to Bill and lastly to me. "When you recognize the amazing work that is being done so we can walk again and see again—and the work we're all doing to defeat NMO—hope wins every time. We will prevail. It is inevitable."

The Power of Rare radiated throughout the room.

Holding back tears, I listened and shifted my focus to where we were all headed next. In that moment I felt almost a surge of energy coming from Ali—connecting with me wordlessly as she so often does—and from all the patients. My daughter and everyone else were getting pumped up, as they urged all of us on toward the finish line.

This year, more than ever before, patients and others in our NMO family had spoken up and spoken out—asking not just what we were doing for them but what more they could do to contribute to our collective cause.

When I thought about it then—as I think about it today—I find the sacrifices and choices to make their struggles meaningful and to find shared purpose more and more extraordinary. When the power of love overcomes fear, great things can be done.

Every year as we come to the end of Patient Day together, we reflect on all that we have that is good. And among our many shared blessings are the caregivers. We have a tradition of taking a special moment to thank them for their sacrifices and to remind them to take care of themselves too. This year, as we did, a spontaneous combination of tears and applause filled the room with a standing ovation.

We have another tradition that usually follows, and that comes from Dr. Yeaman offering a reminder that it's up to all of us to each play our part in solving NMO. He also emphasizes that our ultimate win—the cure—is in each of our patients.

The cure is in the room. It really is. It always has been.

He acknowledges that, yes, it can be overwhelming to imagine how any one patient or any one of us could have something to offer—especially if you think you are alone and powerless—or if others seem to have more options.

So how, then, can any of us choose hope over fear? His answer comes in the form of a personal mantra, adapted from age-old words of wisdom:

Yes, I am only one. But still, I am one.
I cannot do everything. But still I can do something.
And it is precisely because I cannot do everything—
that I must do the something I can do.

At the Power of Rare conference I overheard a newly diagnosed patient tell her mother afterward that she wanted to become involved as an advocate because, "I want to do the something that I can do. And I can."

These moments are ones that are now writing our future, as are some of the other lasting impressions that came out of those three days in March 2017.

Not really "rare"—rather "unique"—in a universe where, in the end, we are all very similar.

—Athos Gianella-Borradori, MD
*Chief Medical Officer, Chugai
Pharmaceutical, in response to
the question "Is each of us rare?"*

PUTTING YOURSELF INTO THE STONE

Revelations often arrive at the least expected of moments. Not unlike the diagnosis of a rare autoimmune disease—or cancer or other life-changing event—that comes out of the blue to radically alter everything in your world, turning it into something you never could have anticipated. Revelations may not always be earth-shattering, but they can hit you in an instant, when you experience their full impact as you might never have done before.

That is what happened for me when I took the stage to deliver my opening remarks at our Roundtable scientific meetings at our 2017 International Roundtable Conference for NMO (our 9th annual)—and our most ambitious and action-packed agenda yet. This year, I was extra-prepared, complete with a PowerPoint slide deck.

For the next two days, and a third day when we would convene Patient Day (our 8th annual), the Power of Rare would be woven into every aspect of the message. The rare work we had done and the rare work to be done would be more than just our conference theme.

But on that morning, even before I said a word, I was reminded again of my cancer scare three years earlier, and how—seemingly more and more every day—we are all facing challenges, disease or otherwise.

No one is immune to having a family member or friend or colleague suddenly given a dire and unexpected prognosis. What I also realized was that the likelihood of being someone or knowing someone with some form of an autoimmune disease is far greater than ever in human history. But then—because no one is immune to the risks—the revelation that hit me was that no one is immune to doing what they can to make a difference. We all have to put ourselves into the healing stone and become part of the cure revolution.

My call to action had to be loud: unless we take brave new steps today, disease will rule tomorrow. My job was clear as I approached the stage.

Yes, the exciting new immune science we have spearheaded—and the blueprint for turning it into cures—matter. Ours is a model for confronting *all* immune-related illnesses, including cancer, infection, heart disease, and other diseases society faces with increasing dread. More and more, evidence is mounting that diseases like Alzheimer's, Parkinson's— perhaps dementia and even the process of aging itself—are consequences of the immune system doing too much or doing too little.

We don't have all the answers yet—but what we do have is a blueprint for collaboration to span the Valley of Death. To transform and improve and save lives.

We have a blueprint to be shared that can be easily applied by emerging leaders in this country and around the world for *revolutionizing how lives can be spared from disease.* Affordable and accessible healthcare, women's and family health, mental health—these are but a few of the great and urgent needs of today and tomorrow. And more than reactive medicine that awaits disease occurrence before action is taken, we must get out in front of disease—through preventive medicine—that foils illness from happening in the first place.

How? It comes back to the reality that no one is immune.

We are not alone in our call to action for change. So I'll ask again: if not all of us, *who?* If not now, *when?*

In less than 10 years, a very short time in the development of new therapeutics, the GJCF has uniquely and proactively brought together top scientists from academia, industry leaders and federal government resources to provide patients with NMO the best chance for effective therapies and the prospect of a cure for this rare disorder.

—Terrence F. Blaschke, MD
Professor of Medicine and Molecular Pharmacology, Emeritus, Stanford University, Palo Alto

A BOLD NEW CURESHOT

Before I came up with my PowerPoint presentation, I'd thought about the great accomplishments of our history when people of good will came together with a sense of urgency to achieve what was called impossible.

In the 1960s, for example, the push to overcome the vast unknowns of outer space, safely set foot on the moon, and return home again became known as the Moonshot. If reaching the moon and conquering the fear of what was still unknown mattered so much to so many, why wouldn't the same be true here on Earth for conquering disease? The stakes were high then and just as high now.

Thinking along those lines, former Vice President Joe Biden is helping spearhead an ongoing and ambitious Cancer Moonshot that I know is going to save and change lives. My hope now is that we can go even further. Beyond the moon. My thought is, *Why not focus on a bolder mission?*—a *Cureshot*: overcoming the mysteries of all human disease, finding safe and effective new ways to prevent and treat them, and returning to health.

My message at our conference was that we could and should be at the forefront of this revolution for cures.

Through NMO, we were zeroing in on the very origins of immune dysfunction in the first place. As Dr. Yeaman always said, we could use the downstream effects in NMO as cellular and molecular breadcrumbs to find the upstream causes. We were exploring potential clues—from genes to germs—and factors that had been underappreciated were getting a second look.

The window of opportunity couldn't be ignored.

The field was changing—from observing the immune system to modifying it. We were talking the language of "omics," from genome to phenome. The world of science and medicine was evolving faster than ever to unravel molecular codes and find patterns in Big Data. We all needed to work this global room.

We were all in a new era—making the leap from toxic chemotherapies to safer biologic therapies. Instead of sledgehammer drugs to wipe out immune systems, molecular forceps of immunotherapies were in hand. We also needed to rewrite the old rules of clinical trials so that a patient who failed one treatment could quickly be moved to another arm of a study to receive a different test drug. We needed to change the world of medicine and make it work for everyone. But that would take more than just us.

And powerful new tools were on the horizon. Even something that once sounded like science fiction, such as "gene editing," was in sight—allowing repair of the very genes that cause disease—making therapy obsolete.

Yet not all this brave new technology was ready for prime-time—which was another reason we needed a collective Cureshot. After all, as Dr. Yeaman reminded us often, the immune system is constantly changing—learning and remembering. So we would need unprecedented solutions to avoid "the snapshot effect," as he called it. Sampling genes or immune systems at only one point in time could be misleading. We needed science and medicine to move at the speed of life.

Certainly, we had much to learn from the Human Genome Project of the twentieth century—and the human microbiome project ongoing.

Those projects were revealing surprises, such as the discovery that each so-called human genome contains a lot of microbial DNA. Curing rare and common diseases alike would require us to understand that *beyond* all the microbes growing in us and on us, their genetic codes are actually *part of us*. Hidden hitchhikers—or even hijackers.

To achieve custom cures, we also needed to know not just what a drug does to a body but also what a body does to a drug. Because even an identical drug can work differently in different people, this would be a key step needed to move beyond one-size-fits-all treatments.

These were only a handful of many obstacles to overcome on our journey to the promised land of personalized and precision medicine. But that day was coming on like a freight train, and we were on board.

That's what I wanted to reinforce with all the members of our NMO community. Yes, our work was daring and we were raising eyebrows—in a good way. How could we up the ante—now more than ever?

The timing gives us a rare opportunity. Rare diseases like NMO are *already* ushering in a new-reality era of medicine. Personal is the new communal. Research into rare has led to new understandings that each person experiences disease through her or his own distinct combination of causes and effects.

Rare diseases are the exceptions that prove the rules.

These opportunities also come with the heavy responsibilities that I believe global leaders must address together. Much more must be done to address the inequality of access to healthcare and to innovative treatments that we're all working toward—and that may be among the most expensive. We know that those with fewer resources are often hit the hardest by illness and will be even more so by the disease pandemics to come. Unless we all invest in taking care of the most in need, progress will be slowed for all in need.

And there are bigger threats to health that can only be solved on a global stage. We have to pay attention to the impact of climate change on the environment and how that could be triggering old and new diseases—rare and common alike.

None of us is immune to taking part in meeting these challenges. No one foundation or organization can do this alone. We all can be inspired and inspire at the same time. We can turn critical health issues that affect us or our loved ones into revolutionary progress for cures. That's what Maria Shriver has done—a role model on many fronts—with her amazing work mobilizing solutions for Alzheimer's.

We have to make our causes personal.

From philanthropists to activists to volunteers—on whatever scale is possible—everyone really does have a role to play.

What is it going to take to solve and prevent diseases—rare and common alike? A global effort and the *will* to do it together. That's our Cureshot.

Not long ago in *Fortune* magazine, I read the three questions that Google X's Astro Teller applies to setting an agenda for any kind of revolutionary shot: 1) Is the problem big enough? 2) Is there a radical solution to the problem? and 3) Is it actually solvable?

There should be no question. From autoimmune disease to cancer, from heart disease to aging, everyone will face a life-challenging medical condition. Immune health *is* the radical solution that must be pursued—and the time is now.

Our global health crisis demands a global response. The problem is big enough. There are even more radical and rare solutions waiting to be applied. It is solvable.

For that to happen, we urgently need enlightened leadership everywhere in the world. How we respond to the health crises of today and those to come will determine whether we prevail or fail. Each of us and all of us.

This could be the great awakening of our time, if we choose to embrace the possibilities. We have the will and the way. We can go further—but not alone.

THE POWER OF DISCOVERY

As I opened our Power of Rare conference, I could appreciate how we had gone from being that little foundation that *could* to the one that *did*. We went from ground zero to becoming a global mover and shaker. Nine years earlier, we had been a small band of revolutionaries—the original Knights of a rare Roundtable—gathered together for a group photo in front of one flag from just one country . . . the United States. At our 2017 conference, there were 175 of the most renowned experts in multiple fields—from neurology to molecular immunology, from drug development to cell-based therapy and so many more. And waving behind me across the back of the stage as I welcomed everyone were twenty-eight different flags. Our very own UN of NMO.

In my imagination, I had always visualized the reality that someday we'd be here with all these flags—symbols of an extraordinary international team—working with us. And now here we were. We had started with the power of love and purpose, and fueled it with courage, faith, and a refusal to accept the status quo.

Center stage was beautifully lit for the delivery of my opening remarks. The moment weighed on me. My intuition told me to move beyond the PowerPoint, so I began to speak from the heart. More my style. A combined sense of urgency and strength filled the air. We had sought to put NMO on the world stage—and now that world was in the room. We had to seize the moment to ask what rare was trying to tell us.

My words flowed out. For me, as I welcomed everyone, it was about what all of us—all working mindful of the same goal—had accomplished so far. It was about applying what we had learned to what remained to be done for patients. It was about the discovery that rare is not so rare, and about the doors and windows NMO was opening to solve even the greatest problems in the world of medicine. And it was about something else that I most wanted to emphasize as I reflected at that moment on all that had been done to get us there—our interconnectedness. It was about doing more together than can be done alone—to discover and share knowledge that will ease human suffering.

The Power of Rare is about drawing a direct line from the personal to the global to the universal.

"When I started this journey," I confessed, "I didn't think I could have found the power in rare . . . I felt really powerless." No longer.

The power we found was from the knowledge that we weren't alone, individually or as a community. Rare mattered to the future, and that gave me strength and a continued resolve to push further to shed light on possibilities that have lived for too long in the dark. I had found power in witnessing the unique and extraordinary abilities in those who joined with us—by necessity or choice—and in their willingness to step up and continually reach further than maybe even they thought they could.

The Power of Rare is the power of discovery. And even more than that—it's the hunger and even obsession to find answers still unknown and apply them to benefit lives.

I took a breath to scan the room and looked into faces of the best of the best—of those who had been on the path with us from the start, and those who were just joining us. What was about to happen for the next two days of our Roundtable sessions would not only alter the future of our living blueprint, but would challenge everyone to review and rethink all that we knew. We would make sure we had missed nothing.

Neither of our keynote speakers were doing work in NMO—but both embodied the Power of Rare. This was clear in my welcome: "I like to think about how others are making discoveries and uncovering secrets from the unknown. We're here to find answers—and I'm bringing outside perspectives to challenge you with questions that haven't been asked before."

On the first day, we heard from Dr. J. Craig Venter, a giant in medical science who literally swam with the sharks to learn from them— and about himself. He may be best known for his work mapping the human genome (and becoming the first human to have his own genome sequenced), as well as being a pioneer of personalized medicine. In his presentation "Human Genomics and the Future of Medicine," Dr. Venter would tell us about the institute he built to promote health and longevity—the largest facility in existence capable of decoding individual genomes to predict and prevent disease. Using supercomputing, he would make his own strong case for how every single disease is distinct and rare. His vision for helping to spur a medical revolution was to make patient care more *proactive* and less *reactive*.

Dr. Venter would note that out of 10,000 individual genomes studied, more than 8,000 presented markers for significantly rare conditions or their risks. This confirmed for me what I felt intuitively—that rare is not only more common than most realize but how few will be *untouched* by rare disease.

On the morning of Day 2, we would hear from Dr. Maria Spiropulu, world-renowned experimental particle physicist and professor from Cal Tech. What could such a person have to do with solving NMO? She was on the team that in 2012 found "the God particle"—the mythical Higgs boson. In her keynote, "The Power of Rare Discoveries," Dr. Spiropulu referenced her own search for rare truths of the universe in dimensions that haven't even been identified. She went on to tell her story of the moment-to-moment series of events leading to proof of the predicted Higgs boson particle. What had been the chances of proving the existence of this "God particle" that held within in it the blueprint for the entire universe? *One in 10 billion,* if you asked her.

How was that even possible to achieve? How could you find something that you believed did exist but couldn't be seen? Citing a parallel to our work to cure NMO, she said the most important breakthroughs came from massively integrated teamwork—and a refusal to ever give up or give in or give way.

Dr. Spiropulu also emphasized how rare has always been critical to every major discovery—reminding us that what we were doing to solve NMO was a model for achieving solutions that can be applied by others.

Dr. Yeaman tied it all together by connecting what Dr. Venter and Dr. Spiropulu—and NMO researchers—had done: not being limited to what could be seen. To that end, he challenged everyone in the room to consider the known and the unknown—the positive and negative space—in human disease. To consider that solving NMO and healing the immune system may have as much to do with the *absence* of molecular and cellular *stop* signs as the *presence* of *go* signs. And if that's the case, how do you look for the absence of a factor? Like the Higgs boson particle, how do you seek an answer that you believe—but have yet to prove? And how could we build that perspective into clinical trials—and fast?

Particles of a new brainstorm to cure NMO were born that day.

WRITING THE NEXT CHAPTERS

Over the next three days, we had a lot of ground to cover. We were aiming for the ultimate mind meld, and we had to open our hearts more than ever. That was the message I most needed to put out there.

"We all know," I reminded everyone, "not a lot of this matters to patients unless NMO can be cured and lifted from their lives. I hear from patients throughout the year: What are we doing? What new progress have we made? The clock is ticking."

We were throwing down the gauntlet to write the next chapters— asking everyone to bring their rarest of capacities to the table. And we were filling the room in a way many said we never could but I had always hoped we would. The drawing Power of Rare was real.

Along with clinicians and researchers, we were now being joined by leaders of academic and medical institutions worldwide. We had nurses and technicians to help us with blood draws—plus industry partners, biotech executives, regulatory agencies, media, venture capitalists, and more. And, of course, patients and their caregivers and loved ones were always front and center.

My main request to everyone in the room was to make sure their rare voices were raised. "I want to continue to hear them—loud," I said, expressing my deepest appreciation. "I want to walk away and think about what new things we've learned and how we can do even better." That would shape our blueprint immediately and most effectively. We would deconstruct every insight as we planned for the future by asking: "What are the remaining challenges? What are the new opportunities?"

These questions were conceived in response to problems that needed solving now—as the greatest discoveries always are. And we needed to put every dollar to the test to achieve even more meaningful results.

For those three days, I listened and processed and observed. Before the experts and patients had arrived, we placed a life-size image of a tree without leaves on one ballroom wall. We offered simple green leaves made of paper for patients and experts alike to use in writing down how they were affected by the Power of Rare—and then invited them to pin their leaves to the NMO Tree of Life. By the time I stood on the stage to thank everyone involved, I looked over and saw a flourishing tree full of messages and insights that we had literally all grown together.

We had come such a long way. I couldn't know ahead of time how we would discover our own God particle of the cure and how to end NMO once and for all. I couldn't see it yet—but I do know it exists.

As I concluded my closing remarks, I brought it all back to the power of love and the power of intention and family—thanking everyone in our community and, of course, Ali and the patients who along with her had just finished their second presentation. And once more, I thanked Bill, who was always there—in the back of the room—never asking to be thanked.

The future was calling. We would move forward with urgency and gratitude as always.

But for now, I want to offer some final thoughts about rare that are most needed in a time when no one is immune to caring and sharing in efforts to face the toughest challenges of our lives.

IT'S NOT ABOUT THE BLUEPRINT

Each of us is one in a billion. Well, one in 7 billion, to be exact—and counting. Each of us is rare. Yet the wonderful irony is that because we all share this fact of being rare, we're not so rare. Each of us—you and I and everyone we love and hold dear—is connected in a healing circle of life-story secrets that can revolutionize the field of medicine and save lives. With or without a dire diagnosis—with or without a cause that directly affects you—you still have the opportunity to use your Power of Rare to make a difference to the world.

As important as it is to have a blueprint for assembling the building blocks of your highest endeavor, in the end it is not about the blueprint. *It's what you do with the blueprint.*

Ask any builder. A blueprint is a piece of paper—flat and lifeless. It guides you to gather the necessary elements and suggests how you can take the important steps for assembling them in a particular order. But it's only two-dimensional. To create three-dimensional, real-world, life-saving change—to become a rare alchemist—it's up to each of us to act on the elements of rare that turn a blueprint into a living, breathing movement.

As I embrace all the aspects and dimensions of rare that have shaped our living blueprint, I admit that when taken individually, none of these capacities are rare at all. What makes for rare power is all of them in their rare combination. Miss one element and the most noble of undertakings is less—the greatest of hope just a wish.

For all those reasons, I share with you my most valued truths about the Power of Rare—that are not so rare—in the sincere hope they will remind you of all that you can do at a time in the world that needs all of us engaged:

VISION. What is it that you believe but doesn't yet exist, and that you desire above all to bring into being? If it is to cure a disease or achieve justice where none has existed, push your rare vision to find your way. Vision can be a lamp in the darkness to guide you through, I promise you.

PEOPLE. Surround yourself with rare and extraordinary and diverse people. Build teams of uncommon movers and shakers who are real-world and real-time innovators. Listen, learn, and empower others to own a stake in the results of your collective efforts. Create incentives for collaboration without eliminating healthy competition. Be open to rare advice that gives you the insight to know the difference between what could be done and what should be done.

PURPOSE. Recognize how your purpose is larger than you and yours. Understand that your leadership role is to problem-solve and take on the biggest challenges one at a time to meet your own goals and those of others. Purpose gives meaning and relevance to all who join with you. Share your rare.

STRATEGY. Rare strategies allow you to ask questions in new ways and to pull from past experiences to create rare innovations. Rare strategies are more about reaching the ends than just creating the means. Always be innovating—as long as there is strong evidence for doing things a new way. Learn from everything you do, whether it succeeds or fails.

MINDSET. Think like a revolutionary and budget like a businessperson to be a practical change maker. Never be afraid of challenging dogma. Have the courage to ask "Why not?" and the strength to accept new perspectives. A rare mind-set allows you to find and apply the wisdom that is hidden in data.

HEART. Last but not least, I must include the power of rare heart—not because I think heart is rare—but because heart is rarely appreciated as an organizing and guiding force for taking on anything as complex as curing a rare disease. Why that is, I'm not sure. What I do know is that the boldest against-all-odds actions require bravery that can only come from heart. Everything we have done to help rare patients and those who love them has begun and ended with heart.

You will not find heart on any chart of the elements or map of the stars. But I know heart exists there—as a capacity to love, give, and care about our fellow human beings at a pure level. Heart connects us spiritually and may be the truest blending of science and faith.

True heart—true spiritual connection—points us in the direction of caring for one another, however and wherever our individual purposes and paths lead us. That is humanity's true north, and it is calling us now more than ever.

We can and we must, all of us, seize this moment to apply what we know to solving the most pressing issues of our time.

That is the gift and the true Power of Rare.

Each one of us is just a visitor to this planet—
a guest—for a limited time.
What greater folly could there be than to spend
this short time alone?
Far better, surely, to use our short time here in
living a meaningful life, enriched by our sense of
connection with others and being of
service to them.
—Dalai Lama

FROM ALI TO MALI

JULY 2017

Every now and then, the universe likes to tap me on the shoulder and re-mind me of the passage of time. Of course, I can do the math. I know it's been a little more than nine years since Ali's eyeball headache appeared out of the blue and made the world seem as if it had stopped spinning on its axis.

But so much has happened so quickly that I keep asking myself, *Wait, how is this possible? Wasn't that just yesterday?* In less than two months Ali will be starting law school. Not that I should be surprised, but I'm still amazed. And whether she ultimately pursues human rights or social justice or another aspect of advocacy, it's not up to me to know how that story will be told. What I do know is that she is thriving, and I live in daily—no, minute-by-minute—*gratitude* that she is.

When we began our journey as a family to take on NMO, it was Ali who inspired the blueprint and helped me find the rare power to bring it to life. I prayed our numbers would grow rapidly and that powerful connections would be made—and that we would become the global com-munity that we are.

When Ali was the one NMO patient we knew, I remember how excited we'd get when our foundation team would report that a patient with
NMO had been located in faraway Africa.

Africa! I'd rush into her room and give her the news. We'd dash down
to my office and put a mark on our Connect the Docs map and thank the
universe that we no longer felt so alone. Well, plenty of those moments
later—through good fortune and good work—awareness of NMO has
spanned the globe. Thousands of NMO cases have now been diagnosed
or are suspected across the African continent.

So much so that two neurologists—Dr. Najib Kissani from Morocco
and Dr. Youssoufa Maiga from Mali—organized the first-ever Pan-
African conference on NMO in 2016. After the success of that conference in Morocco, a second and even more ambitious conference was
planned for summer 2017 in Mali.

Templating our blueprint, the planners began just as we did—by
seeking to get everyone in the room. Urgent goals were set for the Mali
conference. In addition to educating, training, and empowering medical
providers across the continent to better diagnose and treat NMO, the
plans included the creation of an NMO patient and caregiver community
spanning the entire continent.

Mali promised to be a game changer. I was about to learn just how
small the world had become—and in more ways than one.

In a kind of magical twist, Ali reminded me of her time in high
school when she took part in a Model United Nations program. Her
country? *Mali.* She was actually part of the Mali delegation and learned
everything she could about the country so that when her school traveled
to the real United Nations, they could debate policy with knowledge of
the real issues.

The small-world coincidences didn't end there. As it turns out,
Maoloude Touré, a friend and advocate of our foundation, is originally
from Senegal—a next-door neighbor to Mali. While helping with logistics at our Power of Rare conference in Los Angeles, Maoloude connected with Dr. Maiga and heard about plans for the Mali conference.

Afterward, Maoloude—who has no medical or healthcare background—approached me to offer his services.

What would he do? *Everything.* Fluent in five languages—French, English, Arabic, and two native African dialects—he could serve as an all-around translator and, more important, as my representative.

I didn't ask him to undergo a crash course in NMO. But Maoloude insisted he had to learn everything he could to understand more than just the words he was translating. In a matter of days, he read *Saving Each Other*, our Patient Guide, and covered every inch of our website.

Maoloude then translated the *Welcome* speech I asked him to deliver on my behalf into French—the popular language of Mali and one of the two official languages, along with English, to be spoken at the conference. Next, he went to work preparing a PowerPoint to also present at the opening of the conference. He was transporting my Power of Rare message to Africa, blueprint and all.

Maoloude's commitment to be of service to a cause that didn't touch him or his family directly was inspiring to witness. Just to travel to an area impacted by unrest and terrorism was a lot for him to undertake. That, on top of the eighteen-hour flight to Bamako—the capital city of Mali where the conference was being held—would have made it understandable if he opted out. He never considered that.

Maoloude was motivated by heart. This was something he *had* to do—for Africa and for NMO patients everywhere—and because this was the something he *could* do.

Conference registration soon skyrocketed to include 480 attendees, mostly neurologists, from twenty countries. Extraordinary. Among those in attendance would be doctors from Maoloude's native Senegal, Ivory Coast, Benin, Cameroun, Togo, Ghana, Niger, Morocco, Tunisia, Congo Brazaville, RDC Congo, Chad, Mauritania, Guinea Conakry, Gambia, Burkina Faso, Djibouti, Comoros Island, the United States—and, of course, Mali.

Before Maoloude traveled to Mali, I signed several copies of *Saving Each Other* in the hopes they would find their way into the hands of the country's leaders and doctors from the different nations attending the conference. The book would be both a gift of thanks and a wish that they might know how much we cared. When Maoloude arrived in Mali, we started FaceTiming so he could report how much energy and excitement there was around this meeting.

Because this was such an important story of how the blueprint could be applied in new settings and with help from a blueprinter who—like me—didn't necessarily have a medical background, I called on Jesse Dylan to document this Power of Rare story. Somehow Jesse found a camera crew in Kenya who showed up just in time to capture Maoloude's visits to the homes of patients, where he was able to convey my message of hope.

Difficult road conditions required long, slow drives to reach them, often taking hours at a stretch. Where technology allowed, Maoloude would show the video that Ali narrates about the Foundation and then at the end announces, "My name is Ali Guthy, and I have NMO."

What mattered most was that NMO patients and their families in Mali seemed to gain strength from knowing there were people across the oceans who knew their heartache—and were doing all they could to better treat and cure this devastating disease.

If we could find the courage, these patients told Maoloude, so could they.

When Mali's president, Ibrahim Boubacar Keïta, heard about our unique story, he opened doors for Maoloude and others from the conference to speak at the university and local hospitals. And, last not least, the president invited Maoloude and Dr. Maiga to his palace for a reception that included, among other dignitaries, the minister of health and public hygiene, Samba Sow.

The president had not been familiar with NMO before this meeting. He too expressed his surprise that our family, living on the other side of the world, was affected by a disease that citizens in Mali were struggling with. When he learned about the work of our Foundation, President Keïta agreed to support the launch of a new Pan-African Registry for NMO—to be based in Mali.

Maoloude told me that upon receiving the book I had inscribed for him, the president looked at the cover photo and nodded, as if greeting old friends. Then the president, wanting the reassurance of good news that followed, quickly asked, "Tell us, how is Ali?"

Everywhere Maoloude went word had spread about this teenage girl who inspired a rare revolution.

Before long, everyone was asking, "How is Ali?"

Maoloude assured them all that she was doing well and encouraged them also to—as we say—"know more NMO." Echoed by Dr. Maiga, he was able to emphasize the point that the earlier the diagnosis and right therapy, the better the chances for a good outcome.

Watching most every report in real time, I recognized the daunting lack of resources and pressing economic challenges facing most African nations. Still, I loved the global message that NMO doesn't care where you're from or how much money you have. What matters is that we're in this together.

What I had always believed had been proven true: in a smaller and smaller world, the more rare we have in common.

What were the chances of all these connections—2%, 1% percent? I'd say the chances of the rarest of coincidences were closer to 0% I mean think about it. Just six years earlier Ali had presented Mali at the Model United Nations. And now Mali was presenting Ali to all the nations of Africa.

We have come full circle—*from Ali to Mali*—and home again.

All of this was proof—a living validation—that our blueprint could be exported and replicated. There was much to celebrate. But it was also a dedication that there is more to do.

In spite of the amazing advances we have achieved together, for now our community still bears the loss of patients who have become family to all of us. And although they are fewer and fewer, I feel each loss more than ever. For them and all NMO patients and families, I will fight all the harder and push all the further. That's rule one of the blueprint—it's a marathon not a sprint—and I won't stop until there is a cure.

After all the hardship and heartache—after all the brilliance and breakthroughs—we move forward knowing that together we are infinitely wiser and stronger and better. This is *our* story.

What does it mean to have a rare disease? To be alone? To be lost?

Or is there an infinite power in rare?

A decade ago, little was known about neuromyelitis optica. When we learned our daughter had NMO—we felt alone and in the dark.

What began with one mother's love for her daughter has become a global mission for cures. The Power of Rare can help solve the unsolvable—cure the incurable. From rare patients to rare partnerships—we have sparked a bold new movement for health.

The strength of one—raised to the benefit of all—that is *The Power of Rare.*

ACKNOWLEDGMENTS

In the world of makeup, I have always embraced an aesthetic of *less is more*. But when it comes to expressing my most heartfelt love and appreciation to all who have played a part in helping me bring *The Power of Rare* to life, I can only opt for *more*. There just aren't enough words to express how grateful I am.

The truth is that there would never have been a second book to write about our journey to cure NMO if it weren't for all the members of our Guthy-Jackson Charitable Foundation community. I am in constant awe of patients—who are the reason for what we do and who are all my heroes. Thank you for your voices and your advocacy and your strength. You are the cure and you are why we have advanced as quickly as we have. Thank you to caregivers and family members whose sacrifices know no limits.

Dearest Ali, from the moment you made your miraculous appearance in my life, you became my best friend, my closest soul sister, my role model, and my teacher. Over the past ten years, your wisdom, courage, resilience, and rarity have been at the heart of every lesson learned and stride made in the journey we have shared. Whenever I think of your choice to put me into the healing stone for myself, I think of how you do that for countless others everywhere. Thank you for your humor and your light, and for reminding me even in darkness that there is a story yet to be told that ends with a true version of happily ever after.

To each of my three beautiful children—Evan, Ali, and Jackson—I love you with all my heart. Yes, I am also sometimes known as a "smother mother." But hey, that's me. To my wonderful daughter-in-law Tedde, I am so thankful for all you do—and for the joy of my first grandson. You all make me so proud.

And to Bill, my extraordinary, loving husband, for your unconditional support and belief in me—and in all that is possible with love and intention—thank you. At every step of our journey from the moment you toasted to the adventures that lay ahead in our future, you have always been there. Thank you for your great generosity in writing the checks that make our work possible. Thank you for taking the leap of faith as we continue to push past boundaries in our rare approach to a rare disease. Thank you for your vision and insights that elevated the content of *The Power of Rare*.

* * *

I wish to acknowledge—more than he would prefer, I'm sure—Dr. Michael Yeaman, without whom there would be no book. As my coauthor, his generosity of time and brilliance and spirit, and his extraordinary gifts for making the most complex science understandable and relatable, are a blessing to every page. Among the rarest of the rare, Michael is not only one of our original Knights of the Roundtable who chairs our Advisory Board, but his insights into solving NMO have inspired everyone on the team—and are inspiring cures to other diseases as well, autoimmune and beyond. Thank you, Michael, a blueprinter in your own right; I am forever grateful.

To Mim Eichler Rivas—a very, very special and heartfelt thank-you for helping me realize a book that I didn't ever think I'd be able to bring all the words together to write. And you not only helped me find my voice on the page that came along with those words, but you helped bring out the words *and* the heart together to create this book. My thanks come with much love. I am so very grateful.

Thank you, Francine LaSala, for jumping into the mix mid-project to lend your editorial guidance and passion for the material, as well as your wonderful organizational talents.

I am so fortunate my dear friend Loree Rodkin connected me with Judith Regan's rock star publishing production team—with much appreciation for precision under major time constraints to project manager Kurt Andrews. For the beautiful design work, many thanks to Richard Ljoenes and Nancy Singer. Thanks to Alexis Gargagliano for your thoughtful editorial input. And thank you to Hillary Schupf for your PR mastery.

None of these deadlines could have been met nor pages generated without the dedication of everyone on the team at my home office. Much gratitude to all—for keeping me on task and on track, and then some. Thank you, Carl Perkins, for your leadership, your caring, your wisdom, and for always standing shoulder to shoulder with me. Can't be without you. You make rare look easy. A special thank-you to my assistant, Rachael St. Rose for exceptional efforts—from keeping the binders in order through countless drafts to your heart and energy.

Not a day goes by that I don't give thanks to everyone at the offices of the Guthy-Jackson Charitable Foundation. Jacinta Behne, thank you for your guidance and your contributions to the blueprint—and for helping connect us to materials vital to this book. Thank you as well to all the members of the team for your steadfast efforts toward curing NMO and empowering patients—and basically making my life a lot easier—couldn't do it without all of you: Derek Blackway, Daniel Behne, Megan Kenneally, Brian Coords, Renee Rodriguez, and Judy Sheard.

Extra love to my favorite moms—Michelle Dean, Lisa McDaniel, Gabriela Romanow, and so many more—you know who you are.

Katelijn and Filip, your family is in my heart—as is every NMO family—reminding us all why we must move forward bravely and boldly. Always.

And a special thank-you to the Sumaira Foundation for embracing this important work.

To Christine Ha, much gratitude for using your gifts and your voice to raise the volume on NMO. And to everyone on the team from Wondros Global, all my thanks for your vision and artistry in getting the word out about rare.

Writing a chronicle about where we began and where we are today has made me all the more indebted to the work of all of our scientists/clinicians, industry and agency partners, supporters, and allies. A collective acknowledgment to all who have become part of our global undertaking—for devoting your rare brilliance to turning the tide on NMO. To every gifted and devoted team member of the CIRCLES program and all of you around the world who are members of our International Clinical Consortium—thank you for saving lives and making history. Thank you to all the members of our Industry Council and to the leadership and coordinators now at the helm of ongoing clinical trials—with more on the way. Your recognition of the power of rare in NMO patients and your intention to save and improve lives is how we will all win.

I am infinitely grateful to those of you among our original core team members and advisors—aka the Knights of the Roundtable—who have helped inspire *The Power of Rare* from our earliest years. Special thanks to Dr. Katja Van Herle—for being our first champion who gave me hope and her heart, and for her tireless support that has been so critical to everything we've accomplished. Thank you to our stellar GJCF advisors past and present: Doctors Amit Bar-Or, Terrence Blaschke, Michael Clare-Salzler, Terry Smith, Richard Ransohoff, Michael Sofroniew, Andre Van Herle, Howard Weiner, and Michael Yeaman; and thank you to our esteemed consultants, including Doctors Peter Agre, Peter Doherty, James Louie, Jack Simon, Brian Weinshenker, and Dean Wingerchuk.

Among the giants in medicine and science whose names appear in this book—and to whom we are forever grateful—I must add a few more words of appreciation for your part in how we shaped our collaborative model. Sincerest thanks to longtime NMO sleuths and slayers who are at the forefront of better understanding NMO and developing better treatments and cures, including Doctors Brian Weinshenker, Larry Steinman, Angela Vincent, Alan Verkman, Scott Zamvil, Tanuja

Chitnis, Jeffrey Bennett, Michael Levy, Claudia Lucchinetti, May Han, Vijay Kuchroo, Sean Pittock, Anu Jacob, Dean Wingerchuk, Dorland Kimbrough, Jacqueline Palace, Kevin O'Connor, Ben Greenberg, Silvia Tenembaum, Vanda Lennon, Kazuo Fujihara, Friedemann Paul, Jerome DeSeze, Bruce Cree, and so many others around the world. Special thanks to Dr. Nancy Sicotte for your leadership in clinical care and overseeing the Cedars-Sinai NMO conferences that provide vitally needed continuing medical education. I am so grateful to Dr. Najib Kissani from Morocco and Dr. Youssoufa Maiga from Mali for spearheading NMO conferences in Africa. Thank you again to Maoloude Touré, who proved each of us can play a role in improving the lives of patients and curing a disease as rare and complex as NMO.

I want to express special thanks to advisors, investigators and partners who took the time to offer your own take on the Power of Rare and who contributed your words to these pages: Doctors Jeffrey Bennett, Terrence Blaschke, Peter Chin, Athos Gianella-Borradori, Gerald Nepom, Nancy Sicotte, Terry Smith, and Dean Wingerchuk. Thank you to Craig Venter and Maria Spiropulu for sharing your brilliant insights into rare.

Deepest appreciation goes to my generous friends and colleagues who have graciously contributed to this book: Ellen DeGeneres, Gloria Steinem, Maria Shriver, Sherry Lansing, Reese Witherspoon, Tony Robbins, Dustin Hoffman, Arianna Huffington, Jesse Dylan, Greg Renker, and Agapi Stassinopoulos. Further gratitude to experts and dignitaries who provided your eloquence to commend this work: Mali president Ibrahim Boubacar Keïta, Dr. Brian Weinshenker, Dr. Lawrence Steinman, Dr. Robin Smith, Professor Samba Sow, and Professor Mansour Ndiaye.

• • •

Whoever it was who said that bringing a book into the world is a little like giving birth was right. Luckily for me, I have been supported and cheered on in the process by the midwives of my personal sisterhood. For your ongoing circles of healing, thank you to Ellen, Portia, Gloria, Lisa,

Robin, Julie, Janice, Kathy, Sherri, Pam, Lynn, Loree, and Olivia, and each of you who have contributed to my life lessons that have informed the chapters of this book.

These thanks would not be complete without special recognition of additional family members who have been gifts in my 2% life. Thank you to my mom, who taught me long ago that when the going gets rough, to dry my tears, wash my face, put on my makeup, and get out there. Much appreciation to my sister Audrey, my niece Nicole, and siblings Andrea, Danny, and Mark. Love always to the North Carolina Guthy family—with endless gratitude for being part of the journey to cure NMO.

Blessings and thanks to those loved ones who are no longer here and are deeply missed—but who continue to send me strength and purpose from above.

On behalf of Bill and me, and our extraordinary foundation team, we offer special thanks to all who have and will continue to join us on our journey. We will honor and never forget the memories of each person who has been part of our extended family and has been lost to NMO. We will stand and advocate for all patients facing this disease. We will continue to champion the life-saving brilliance of the best and the brightest in science and medicine who have committed their highest capacities to our cause. We will steward even more effective connections among academia, industry, and regulatory partners. We will push past all barriers on the fast track to discovering life-saving therapies and cures. We will lead in unraveling the mysteries of immune dysfunction and share what we learn with all in search of answers.

We do this for our daughter—and all the daughters and mothers, sons and fathers, families and friends, who live with NMO and other illnesses. We do this too for the millions more who may be helped by our work—and hopefully by yours too.

> With love, faith, and gratitude always,
> Victoria

RESOURCES

To learn more about NMO, our rare approach to this rare disease, how you can make a difference, and the multitude of resources ready for access, the **NMO Resources Smartphone App** is available for free download at digital app storefronts and at www.guthyjacksonfoundation.org/nmo-apps-software.

You are also invited to visit The Guthy-Jackson Charitable Foundation website to explore all things NMO:

www.guthyjacksonfoundation.org

Some of our most frequently accessed links include:

FEATURED VIDEOS

The NMO Story
    https://guthyjacksonfoundation.org/videos/the-nmo-story

Ali Guthy and The Guthy-Jackson Charitable Foundation
    https://guthyjacksonfoundation.org/videos/ali-guthy-and-the-guthy-jackson-charitable-foundation

Pioneering a New Scientific Research Model

> https://guthyjacksonfoundation.org/videos/pioneering-a-new-scientific-research-model

SAVING EACH OTHER & RECOMMENDED READING

To order *Saving Each Other: A Mystery Illness—A Search for a Cure—A Mother Daughter Love Story* by Victoria Jackson & Ali Guthy—and view a list of recommended and related books:

https://guthyjacksonfoundation.org/recommended-reading

FREQUENTLY ACCESSED INFORMATION

About NMO

> www.guthyjacksonfoundation.org/neuromyelitis-optica-nmo

NMO Diagnosis

> www.guthyjacksonfoundation.org/diagnosis

NMO FAQs

> www.guthyjacksonfoundation.org/nmo-faqs

How NMO Clinical Trials Work

> www.guthyjacksonfoundation.org/clinical-trials

NMO Patient Resource Guide (3rd Edition)

> https://guthyjacksonfoundation.org/tools-for-download

NMO/MS: What You Need to Know Brochure

> https://guthyjacksonfoundation.org/tools-for-download

Multiple Sclerosis & NMO

> www.guthyjacksonfoundation.org/multiple-sclerosis-nmo

CIRCLES NMO Biorepository Study
www.guthyjacksonfoundation.org/blood-bank

Spectrum Library
www.guthyjacksonfoundation.org/spectrum

NMO TV
www.guthyjacksonfoundation.org/album/featured-videos

VOICES OF NMO: PATIENT STORIES

NMOtion Blog
https://guthyjacksonfoundation.org/blog

NMO Diaries
www.nmodiaries.com

Patient H69
https://patienth69.com

Sumaira Foundation "Voices of NMO"
www.sumairafoundation.org/voices-of-nmo

Tattered Edge Blog
www.tatterededge.blogspot.com

HOW YOU CAN DONATE TO THE CURE

None of us can solve NMO alone. As we expand our fund-raising capacities with the creation of The Guthy-Jackson Research Foundation, Inc., we welcome donations from public, private, government, and commercial organizations, as well as donations from fund-raising events, families, friends, and individuals like you. One hundred percent of all donations are appropriated directly to NMO research. Please consider making a tax-deductible contribution on our website's *Donate* page: https://guthy-jacksonfoundation.org/donate

Thank you for all you do.

RELATED NMO RESOURCES

American Autoimmune Related Diseases Association, Inc.
   https://www.aarda.org

Autoimmune Centers of Excellence
   http://www.autoimmunitycenters.org

The Blind Cook
   www.theblindcook.com

Clinical Trials Database (search "Neuromyelitis Optica")
   www.clinicaltrials.gov

French Cohort and Biobank for NMO (NOMADMUS)
   http://www.edmus.org/en/studies/devic_general.html

Genetic and Rare Diseases Information Center
   https://rarediseases.info.nih.gov/diseases/6267/neuromyelitis-optica

German Neuromyelitis Optica Study Group (NEMOS)
   https://nemos-net.de/english-summary.html

Global Genes
   https://globalgenes.org

Invisible Disabilities Association
   https://invisibledisabilities.org

Johns Hopkins NMO Clinic
   www.nmoresearch.org

National Center for Advancing Translational Sciences at NIH
    Genetic and Rare Diseases Information Center
    https://rarediseases.info.nih.gov/diseases

National Center for Advancing Translational Sciences at NIH
    Genetic and Rare Diseases Information Center / NMO Homepage
    https://rarediseases.info.nih.gov/diseases/6267/neuromyelitis-optica

National Center for Biotechnology Information
    www.ncbi.nlm.nih.gov/pubmed

National Institute of Neurological Disorders and Stroke
    www.ninds.nih.gov

National Institutes of Arthritis and Musculoskeletal & Skin Diseases
    Autoimmune Diseases Homepage
    https://www.niams.nih.gov/health_info/Autoimmune/default.asp

National Institutes of Health
    www.nih.gov

National Multiple Sclerosis Society
    www.nationalmssociety.org

National Organization for Rare Disorders
    https://rarediseases.org

NMO–UK Rare Illness Research Foundation
    http://nmo-ukresearchfoundation.org

NoMOre! NMO
    www.nomorenmo.com

Rare Disease Day
    www.rarediseaseday.org

Rare Disease Report
www.raredr.com

Sumaira Foundation for NMO
www.sumairafoundation.org

Transverse Myelitis Association
https://myelitis.org

FACEBOOK ONLINE NMO SUPPORT GROUPS

Devic's Fighters
www.facebook.com/groups/112799285465693

My Devic's Family
www.facebook.com/groups/MyDevicsFamily

NMO: Our Fight for a Cure
www.facebook.com/groups/742460559139453

NMO Spectrum UK Community
www.facebook.com/groups/189082381161844

NMO/SD Support Australia (Neuromyelitis Optica)
www.facebook.com/groups/devicsdiseasenmosupportgroupaustralia

Of course, all of these resources comprise only a partial list of what's available. Please stay connected.